CLOSE TO MY HEART

The Terrifying, Sometimes Humorous
Journey to a Double-Lung Transplant

By

Robert Emmet

D1260063

Close to My Heart: The Terrifying, Sometimes Humorous Journey
to a Double-Lung Transplant
By Robert Emmet
© Copyright Robert Emmet, 2020

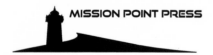

MISSION POINT PRESS

Mission Point Press
2554 ChandlerRoad
Traverse City, Michigan 49696
www.MissionPointPress.com

ISBN: 978-1-950659-52-4
Library of Congress Control Number: 2020906745

Printed in the United States of America

For Jacqueline, Zachera, and Ryan

Acknowledgements

Although I've agreed to guard the identities of the many medical professionals who helped me come back to life, I want to share my appreciation. So "thank you." You know who you are.

There are also some special people who assisted in my recovery and the publication of this book, whom I can mention:

My incredible wife Jackie, daughter Zachera, and Ryan, who stood by me.

The unending support of Boyne City, Michigan, and our close group of friends who take care of each other.

Dr. Michael Harmeling, who started my path to recovery and is a wonderful friend.

Boyne Resorts, Steve Kircher, and Ed Grice whose backing and sponsorship brought this book to fruition.

Jennie Moody and Julie Schmittdiel – two great friends in the science and medical field who first reviewed and critiqued Close to My Heart to assure that my recollections were generally true and made sense.

Contents

Section Two: POST

Introduction

To those who helped me through my transplant and put up with a myriad of rants and raves—thank you. There were many.

As normal days flow by, most of us don't focus on organ donation. We don't walk around thinking about needing a body part or what would happen if we got hurt or dangerously sick. I know I didn't. Hopefully this book will shed an enormous spotlight on organ donors. A percentage of profits from this book is being donated to the Pulmonary Fibrosis Foundation and Lung Transplant Patient & Family Assistance Fund, both of which help transplant patients while they are enduring one of the most difficult times of their lives.

Many chapters in this book will open with my wife Jackie's words—in *italics*...ending with a "Jac." These are thoughts and feelings she logged in her journal during my transplant recovery. These excerpts were added because they offer a glimpse, a window, into how Jackie helped me survive and how she made it through as well.

Foreword

Boyne Mountain Resort is a proud sponsor of *Close to My Heart*.

Robert Emmet, the book's author and a longtime teacher at Boyne City Public Schools, helped shape the lives of many families within Boyne Mountain's neighboring community, Boyne City. He also greatly influenced the lives of Stephen Kircher, president and CEO of Boyne Resorts, and the general manager of Boyne Mountain Resort, Ed Grice.

Established in 1949, Boyne Mountain recently surpassed 70 years of providing skiing and riding opportunities in northern Michigan. The resort started with one of America's first chairlifts—still in operation today—and now offers a range of services: lodging, dining, spa, year-round outdoor recreation, and Michigan's largest indoor waterpark, Avalanche Bay.

The growth of Boyne Mountain would not have been possible without the time, energy, and heart from many members of the community. Working with Robert on his new book was the resort's opportunity to give back.

We're proud to note that part of the proceeds of *Close to My Heart* will benefit the Pulmonary Fibrosis Foundation and Lung Transplant Patient & Family Assistance Fund.

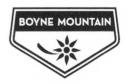

Dad,

I'm sitting on the floor of the hotel room. Mom and Ryan are asleep, and you went into surgery for a double-lung transplant about two hours ago. I'm too scared to sleep, so I decided to write you a letter because these words are for you, and that means you will have to wake up and read them.

Our relationship is unique because we see each other as whole people, not just in our roles to one another. You never made stupid jokes about bringing home a boyfriend and never called me your little princess. You treated me as a whole individual during every stage of my life. I always felt respected and if I had something to say, I was taken seriously, which is one of my favorite things about being your daughter.

My whole life, I never let the thought in that one day I will lose you. Partially because I thought I had many years before that kind of thought was necessary, and partially because I convinced myself that day would never come. You and Mom created a life for me that was so safe and free of worry, I never stopped to think what it would be like without the two of you supporting me. IPF changed all that. This past year of testing, bad medical news, and more tears than we've ever shed, has been miserable. Every time I think about how hard it's been on Mom and me, I remember how compounded that is for you. The one who's being poked, pushed, and scanned—the one who's coughing...and coughing. It must have been so challenging at times just to keep going. I know in my heart you're doing all this for Mom and me. You've made your life about making us happy and it's never been more evident than during the last six months. So, thank you.

Thank you for every pill, shot, stitch, test, probe, discomfort, and difficult breath. Thank you for being brave enough to go into that operating room. Thank you for fighting to give us more time together. Thank you, Dad, for "raging against the dying of the light."

– Zachera

Preface

Doctors in northern Michigan told me I would die by Christmas. My computerized tomography (CT) scan indicated idiopathic pulmonary fibrosis (IPF) had already honeycombed the bottoms of both of my lungs and was matriculating upward, choking off my lungs' ability to process oxygen. The impermanence of our lives is not daytime TV. My existence was shaken and uprooted.

On Feb. 19, 2016, a ten-hour double-lung transplant operation was performed on me by incredible humans who placed another person's lungs into my chest. What happened is about doctors, nurses, staff, and patients all blending together into an amazing cacophony...a story needing to be told. They are all important, their stories are important, their lives are precious.

Trying to write about the whole endeavor was tricky. My immediate problem: subject material. Who wants to read a book about massive surgical procedures, catheters, needles, tubes, bedpans, and buckets? Don't even ask about buckets. Even if this book could actually help people, how to coerce someone to read it? Not exactly beach material.

But—the infamous "butt"—what if my writing described positive and funny things that happened along the way, including: organ donors, incredible surgeons, Garrett's Chicago Style Caramel Corn, walkers, frozen soup, and exceptionally tough patients surviving against all odds? True stories swirling around me daily all at once...crazy, hilarious, massively difficult, zany, and sometimes immensely sad. A journey through a double-lung transplant could help someone else heading into the same harsh realities on the brink of their scariest days.

My hospital counselor Paul asked, "Ever think about writing a book about your experiences? You taught English, right?"

My answer: "Well...who in the world would want to read it? It wasn't pretty, you know." We laughed. The staff knew all too well.

"Robert, what you have to say could help someone in the same shoes. Hardly anyone has written a book about going through a double-lung transplant. There are plenty of medical journal articles written in doctor speak, but hardly any from an actual patient."

Skeptical, I offered, "Ok...two things. One: Writing a book isn't something one does on a lark ...and...two: I have no iota where to start (strange word, "iota"). It won't be easy to read, it'll be tough stuff, there will be swearing because...well...there was. A lot of it!"

Paul sat back in his chair. "You'll figure it out. You have lots to say."

Six months later Paul asked me, again, to seriously consider it. Now, a year and a half after my transplant, I mulled it over. Even published, would it sit on a dusty bookstore shelf with a pic of me in some cheesy sport coat pleading, "Buy me! Surgery stuff! Nasty but fun!" As if some girl chewing gum would say to her hulk boyfriend parked at the mall in his jacked-up Ram 1500 with balls hanging from the hitch, "Hey, hon, let's go back in and buy that cool transplant book!" Camera take of boyfriend revving engine, hysterically laughing, and peeling out. It's just how I felt...guess it wouldn't be that bad...I mean...Mr. Big Truck probably doesn't read...well, much...I don't know.

Early on I told Paul, "I'll do anything to help after the way all of you took care of me." So, there was that, plus he was right; helping would be important. I had never written a book, but I'd never had a double-lung transplant either.

Paul and I made a plan. First, I would meet some of his patients who were heading into a transplant. The proposal also involved my promise to start writing. It didn't take long before a meeting was set up and chapter one began.

One of Paul's "pre" patients was Josh. Approaching our hospital meeting area, I saw Josh was in a wheelchair pulled up close to a cafeteria table in Mercy Mercy Hospital Mother Mary Mercy's (MMHMMM) food court. He looked slightly younger than me, graying hair, and was all hunched up with his head down. Josh's wife, Dana, was sitting next to him. She was fairly short, around sixty years old, had a cute blond bob, and was wearing a bright-colored, flowery A-line dress. She stood up and greeted me with a warm smile, thanking me for taking the time. You could see in her eyes she was trying with all her might to be positive for her husband.

I introduced myself and Dana said, "Paul, the lung transplant team's counselor, told us you would be able to speak with us. Do you know Paul?"

"Yes, I do," I answered. Josh didn't say anything, just kept looking down at his knees. Explaining my transplant was a year ago, I was about to discuss my experience when Josh looked up as if to say something, but stopped. I knew why. I had been right there.

Josh's eyes welled up and he started crying. He was completely overwhelmed. Taking hold of his arm, I said, "You can do this." I had barely met him, but the thing was, he was so mortified, so scared by what was happening to him, "hello" wasn't even possible.

That day, it became clear discussing medical aspects with a patient was totally a doctor's job. Where I could help was assisting with the unknown, a patient's deep, deep fear. Josh was heading into scary territory—ground he knew nothing about. Once Dana began to describe what they had been through so far, Josh started to calm down. His hands loosened their grip. He sat up in his chair and began asking questions I knew came from the bottom of his anguish. Some of my answers made Josh look at Dana as if what they thought was pure dread might not be quite as bad—as if surviving a lung transplant was actually possible. We talked about my new routine: biking an hour a day, doing most things I used to do. The living-proof thing. Again, looking straight in Josh's eyes, I said, "I felt hopeless at first, but now I have my wife Jackie, and my family. I know you can truly do this." Dana started to cry, but kept Josh from seeing her. We took our time and had a good lunch together.

As for my book, where to start? First, I made up fictional names for everyone because confidentiality is imperative. I'd love to tell you about each person who aided me through tough times, long nights, and hospital food...but I can't. They're in this book, they'll recognize the moments, but privacy —as in the song "Grease"— "is the word."

Second, my daughter Zachera told me to create three goals for my book. I decided my first goal was to highlight organ donors. Second, to spotlight the incredible work doctors and staff accomplish every day at major hospitals. Third, to present how loving support by family and friends can bring someone back into this world. Soon my pages began to paint humorous and lighthearted instances. That said, it was imperative readers knew some patients along the way endured far more difficult times than I experienced. My personal transplant journey was icing on all sides of a cake— incredibly lucky. Many patients didn't fare the same. A lung transplant, any transplant, or major surgery is an incredible feat and many patients are brought back to life. But sometimes they die. How immense.

Here's the thing: These words represent an intense undertaking. Patients surrounding me in MMHMMM's lung transplant department were by far the strongest, toughest, heroic people I've ever met. Yes, we laughed together. Funny stories actually helped us get through it all one way or another. Sometimes we cried together, which was exceptionally hard, but patients did what they had to do to keep going.

"Keep on keeping on" was the credo by which each patient started their day. Whether it was my family—Jackie, Zachera and Ryan and their little dog Oliver—who wove their way through my surgery and recovery, or the woman in the next room who had been hospitalized for three straight months, the will to never give up surrounded me. It was the only way.

Please don't go all *Great Expectations* on me—this was all Paul's idea! I swear. I'm blaming the whole thing on him. What happened along my journey is as remembered. That's saying a lot considering my large "basket" of meds, which at one point totaled thirty-seven pills a day. It was so crazy, so insane, it's amazing I even remember trash day! Due to all of this, (and the meds), I've explained what happened in the best way I could (the meds). Sometimes thoughts come streaming out of my head from different directions all at once.

Because days were exceedingly bizarre, I tried to reflect the same here, so you could get the hang and experience it too…LOL…Ok, notttt, but…My tangents are directly related to the equation $Y = MX+B2$ GGH, which translates to "meds taken by right-brained, now irrational person." Life became erratic with a side salad. It was loud, happy, hard, clangy, wet, introspective, spongy, chaotic, sad, strangely quiet, blurry, slim shady, and weird. If that makes sense, then…you get it.

For an average person like me, my transplant journey was more than amazing. Amazing from the moment I couldn't breathe riding my bike…to a day in our boat.

ONE

PRE

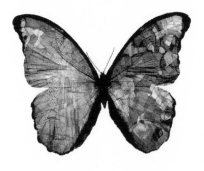

1

One Fine Day

One of the best weather months of the year in northern Michigan is September. It's a well-known secret to us locals living year-round in these parts because all the summer tourists take their last look, lick their last cone, perform their last trunk slam, and steer their way back downstate at the end of August. Most never experience what it's like here in early fall. Also, like clockwork, just as the kids head back to school the day after Labor Day, power up their new Notepads, iPads, GooGits, BlipBlops, or just plain spiral notebooks, don their sport jerseys / band uniforms / helmets / soccer cleats, and take their student council seat—we have brilliant, sunny, 80- to 85-degree days. It rains a lot in late August up here, but come September, it's warm and beautiful.

I'm sure you have a place you love. A time and place to get away from everything. A place you daydream about at work when stress is coming out of your pores. This particular fall day was like that. Our fall season no longer included jet skis howling back and forth by the edge of the beach, potbellied beer drinkers blasting country music on boom boxes, and kids screaming at their parents for being ignored. All that cacophony packed up and disappeared south down the I-75 corridor like circus wagons to places like Grand Rapids, Detroit, Chicago, and Columbus.

It's important you know what happened on this day because it changed our lives. My wife, Jackie, always had a tough time teaching her first graders on early fall days because after a born-free summer they weren't ready to settle down. Adding to the fray was the surprisingly warm weather and the fact that Jackie's elementary classroom didn't have air conditioning. After a long day getting her fidgety, sweaty first-graders to remember where their seat was and that lunchtime wasn't five minutes after school started, Jackie was more than ready to come home, go for a run in the woods, and then quietly relax on our boat.

Occasionally, during this time of year with Lake Charlevoix glistening, Jackie and I would take our 23 ft. Regal out and motor around Old State Park Point to an area called Glenwood Beach—a great spot to swim either from off the back of the boat or from the beach because of the large sandbar running along the shoreline of the park. The beach is known by residents as one of the most serene spots on Lake Charlevoix—a twenty-two-mile-long lake extending from Boyne City on the east end, Charlevoix on the west, with a south arm to East Jordan. Boats anchor on the edge of the drop-off at Glenwood Beach and enjoy the pure sand bottom and clear aqua water. You can literally see the bottom all the way to shore, with a view that includes a bird sanctuary nesting area for ospreys and tall dark-green pine trees creating a mirrored painting of northern Michigan.

Glenwood Beach's sandbar goes quite a ways out into the lake until the depth drops from four or five feet to twenty-five feet quickly. Local swimmers are aware of the drop-off because the water changes color from light blue to navy, signifying the edge. There's even a posted warning sign. Even if you did slip into the deeper water, you could simply swim back to the sandbar.

On this stunning fall day, Jackie and I pulled our boat out slowly from our dock and meandered around the point, anchoring at the edge of the Glenwood Beach sandbar as we always did. It was easy to set an anchor because of the sandy bottom, and provided just the right depth to get in the shallow water off the stern platform. Once settled, we put up our portable blue canopy for shade and attached the canopy's bungee cords to half-moon cleats mounted on the port and starboard sides. The sun's rays were strong, so the canopy's shade made it just right for lying in the warmth, or taking a plunge into the cool, clear water. Of course, munchies, wine, quiet reading, and nodding off were part of the plan. A medium breeze was about, and waves lapped against the side of the boat.

Later in the afternoon, the wind started to pick up some, as it always did on Lake Charlevoix due to the difference between the warm land and the cool water. As the wind puffs got stronger, our canopy started billowing, making a light popping sound. Waking up from the third time through the same paragraph of my book, I looked over at Jackie, who was also just about asleep from the intoxicating slow rocking of the boat, and said, "You know, we should probably take the canopy down. The wind is picking up."

Jackie murmured, "It'll be fine. Don't worry about it."

"What?" I asked.

"It's not going anywhere," she said, closing her eyes.

I grudgingly agreed and continued reading. Ten or fifteen minutes later, a large gust of wind made the canopy pop louder and pull hard on the elastic cords. I ignored it, until it happened a third time.

"We're going to lose the canopy if we leave it up," I said.

Jackie sat up slowly and said, "Allllrightttt, you're probably right. Let's take it down. It's just so nice lying here."

"I know, but..."

Just as I was speaking, a larger blast of wind hit us, and the canopy looked like it was going to rip in half. We immediately jumped up and commenced taking it down. We knew the routine, but the strong wind was making things more difficult than normal. When we tried to unclip the bungees from the sides of the boat, the entire canopy let loose. Pieces started flying everywhere. I grabbed the main metal section to avoid being hit, and Jackie lunged to catch the long plastic stays now sliding out of their canopy sheaths. She got all but one, which bounced down towards the back of the boat, rolling slowly towards the edge of the stern. I couldn't let go of the metal post in my hands, and Jackie was trying to save the canopy from flying away. We tried to quickly put everything down and reach for the stay, but it kept rolling, hit the swim platform below, and dropped into the lake.

Normally, this wouldn't have been a problem. We were anchored, the bottom of the lake off Glenwood Beach was sandy, and the stay would just be lying on the bottom in five feet of water or so. Since the stay was white, it would be easy to see. We grabbed the rest of the canopy, wrapped everything up, and slid it all back in its storage bag. Jackie stowed it in our small cabin as I knelt on the stern seat peering into the water.

Since we were anchored and had a fairly long rode out, our boat was slowly swinging in a large arc as the wind shifted directions. At one point during its arc, our boat would be out over the deep water. On the alternate swing, we were only in four or five feet of water. The errant plastic stay fell near the edge of the drop-off, but only in what looked like a depth of eight feet or so.

Leaning over the side, I could see the long white image on the bottom, and yelled to Jackie as she came up from below, "The stay that came out is right there. I can see it. It's out there…just lying on the bottom. I'll dive down and get it!"

Jackie, now kneeling beside me, wasn't so sure. "I don't know. Looks kind of deep."

This wasn't the first time we had dropped something in the water through our boating years. We had retrieved many items in shallow water: dropped tools, a watch, all the things that can easily roll and slide off a boat. "It's right there. I can get it."

Jackie said, "Ok, but be careful."

"Piece of cake," I said, peeling off my shirt and gingerly stepping out on the swim platform. Being a swimmer all my life, retrieving the stay was a minor task at best. Funny how we think and expect everything in life to keep going on a normal, straight continuum. At that moment, having some type of dangerous lung disease was the furthest thing from my mind. Since summer allergies came and went each year, my nagging breathing issue seemed like no big deal, just that—allergies. So what if I coughed here and there, got fatigued once in a while. That's what happens to everyone when they get older, right? We do what we always do...until we can't.

Taking one last look in the clear blue water to see exactly where the stay was, I dove in. The brisk water hit me like a slap. Lake Charlevoix warmed up to a pleasant temperature during the summer, but once fall arrived, it was cold. I surfaced and, shivering, yelled out, "Wowwww! Huuuuuffff...that'ssss...wow...wayyyy cold!!"

While I was treading water, Jackie laughed, no doubt thinking I was making a bigger fuss than necessary. Vigorously slapping my arms to get used to the cold temperature and kicking my legs, I tried to hover over the spot where the white plastic canopy stay sat on the bottom. The stay's image was shimmering, seemingly moving because of the waves. Like it was old hat, I immediately dove downward, kicking hard, and pulling water behind me with my hands and arms. Halfway down, I realized the stay was in deeper water than it appeared. Depth was always deceiving in water, so I turned around and swam back up to the surface for more air. I heard Jackie yell, "Not worth the trouble. We'll get another one at West End Marine."

I insisted, "No, I can get it. It's right there." Sputtering water, I shouted to Jackie, who was still watching my antics, "It's...deeper... sppplllssss...than...I thoughtttt...I'll get it this time!"

Jackie yelled back, "Come on, forget it!"

"It's ok," I said, water splashing. "It's right there. Almost got it the first time!" Turning to look down to make sure the stay was right below, I took a big, long gulp of air and dove down, kicking and pulling hard. This second time I had more power downward and was just about to grab the stay when something inside my body hit me. Something was wrong. Way wrong. My chest hurt. I was in deep water and out of air! My lungs weren't working. I had done this so many times before and nothing like this had ever happened. Panicking, I looked up and saw the surface above me. *Gotta get up fast, don't know what's happening.* My lungs were collapsing. Nothing was right. My arms and legs wouldn't move and had no strength at all. Somehow, I burst to the surface. My body wasn't responding, no oxygen, all gone. With my lungs aching, I tried to flail my arms as best I could to stay on top of the water. I screamed to Jackie, "Help!...Can't make it! Help me!"

Through my water-filled eyes, Jackie's image was yelling something back—couldn't hear—slipping back down. "Hlpppp!...me!!"

Jackie immediately turned and grabbed something in the boat. Water was running down my nose and mouth. I blew it out, but more came in. I was gagging and couldn't breathe. My legs wouldn't move. No oxygen, the feeling was overtaking me. Everything was closing in. Yelling again, "Hlpppp...not...make...!!" Gurgling "Hlpppp!" my body slipping downward, I knew I was drowning and couldn't stop it. Time was in slow motion. Stopping. A vivid, clear thought at that very moment came upon me—*I'm drowning and I'm going to die.* Everything getting slower. Alarms flashing in my brain: *Can't be happening. Can't be happening.*

I have no idea how, but I got to the surface one last time. Through the splashing water, Jackie was throwing something towards me. Something white landed...nothing left...lurched out towards the image...last gasp...hand hit...held on...Jackie had grabbed a dock line, instantly tied it to a floatation cushion lying on a seat, and, holding on to one end as we had practiced, threw the cushion out towards me as far as she could. A perfect pitch.

How Jackie tied the dock line to the cushion so fast, coiled it, and threw it out perfectly to me I'll never, never know. A one-time throw. It had to be. No seconds left...incredible.

Throughout my life, Jackie always came through when it counted. Always. She only had time for one throw, one try. When she saw my hand grab ahold of the top of the cushion, she started pulling me towards the boat. It took all my strength to hang on, water still going down my nose, the cushion holding me up. Air! My hands were cramping...tried to get my arm up on top of the cushion but couldn't...started slipping back down...but with precious oxygen I was able to kick and hold on.

A long way from safe, Jackie pulled me towards the boat as fast as she could. As I got close, I reached up with one hand to take a stab at the flagging swim ladder, but missed and slipped back down, hitting my mouth on the swim platform. All I remember was the boat bobbing everywhere, the waves splashing water all around me, and Jackie trying to reach me. I tried to hold on to the cushion as long as I could, kicking and kicking to stay afloat. Blood was everywhere. Jackie frantically laid down on the swim platform, forced her arm under my arm, and held me against the back of the boat that was slamming up and down. She gave me a chance for more air. Hanging against the swim ladder and platform, the sharp ladder's edge cut into my arm; it didn't matter. I was breathing and wasn't going to drown—thanks to Jackie.

My chest was heaving, burning, but I could feel precious oxygen moving back into my body, energy surging slowly through me like it was alive. Breathing, breathing oxygen. Jackie held tight. Finally, we tried to get me around to the swim ladder to find a rung. I pulled my left foot up to the first rung, but missed and fell back. Jackie couldn't hold me because the boat was bobbing, and I was twice her size. I hung desperately to the ladder with one hand as we both tried to catch our breath. After a few minutes, with air and Jackie's help, I grabbed the edge of the swim platform, got the ball of my foot set firmly on a ladder rung, nodded to Jackie, and she pulled up as hard as she could to get my chest and arms up on top of the platform. Bleeding, my arms trembling from exhaustion, I was halfway up on the platform with my legs dangling. I didn't want Jackie to know my shaking was from fright. I didn't want Jackie to know what I knew and felt. How it was over—how close her saving me had been.

But she knew. Another second and I would have died. Jackie's perfect throw—a Willie Mays over-the-head catch—or I would have drowned.

Struggling to get me from the swim platform and onto the deck of our boat, Jackie saw the cut on my side was bleeding considerably. She grabbed a towel and held it tight against the flow of blood. Watery blood ran all over the cabin. We both just sat there as the birds quietly dried their wings on the edge of the beach and the afternoon waned under a beautiful sky. No one there knew what had just happened. People walked up and down the beach, kids threw a ball back and forth.

When I yelled for help and slipped below the water's surface, Jackie would never have been able to jump in, swim to where I went under, find me, and somehow pull me to the surface. I would have died. At the moment it was happening, I was slipping away, ending, and the most important person in my world saved me.

We looked at each other in silence. Finally, Jackie said, "Let's go home, ok?"

"Yep," I said.

We went through the motions of cleaning up. We laid wet towels on the back of the seats to dry, and put the bloody ones in a bag to take home. Jackie started the boat, slid it in gear, and pulled slowly forward as I shakily knelt on the bow, gathering in the anchor line. Once the anchor was stowed, I carefully made it back into the cabin and Jackie drove back to our dock.

We didn't say much. Jackie didn't like to pull into our hoist, and asked me to take the wheel as I always did. I didn't do very well. I was still shaking. The boat, which was used to sliding in quietly, clanged its way into our slip, and Jackie held onto the hoist, steadying us until the engine was off. We put things away, Jackie took her beach bag, and we snapped the boat cover down.

Walking down the dock, we both knew how close it had been. We were both upset. We had heard about people drowning for years, how fast it can happen, how easily someone can get themselves in trouble. But, like most people, we never thought it would happen to us. Now it had happened, except I didn't drown. I was alive.

Not sure if you ever noticed, but when accidents happen, it's slam bang, over. There never seems to be conscious thought. If asked about it, people say, "I don't know, it just happened out of the blue." Maybe it depends on the situation, but on that particular day, I was completely aware. Aware of everything. Of vivid, full conscious thought. Time suspended as I dropped down below the water's surface. My life light was going out, and I was watching it happen.

Before all this took place, I had no idea my lungs were so badly damaged. There was always an excuse for my body's shortcomings. Accepting something was wrong didn't happen—"It'll go away. I'm just getting older. Allergies, nothing serious." You know the drill—don't let the truth in—until that afternoon. As Jackie and I walked slowly down the path to our home, my lung transplant journey had started.

2

An Incredible Journey…
in Homage to the Movie…

The next morning during breakfast, after putting those frightful hours somewhat behind us, Jackie looked at me from across our kitchen table. I knew it was coming; it needed to. She said, "Yesterday was scary." Her beautiful eyes welled up.

I didn't say anything at first. The raw fact of the matter—it was extremely scary. When life throws an exceedingly dangerous moment, sometimes there's a fine, fine line between living or dying. A much finer line than all of us think. If an instant had been slightly different, somewhat off, I wouldn't have made it. A second in time, a shorter throw, a missed grab, and Jackie would have been dealing with a horrible, horrible situation—alone. All alone trying to call an ambulance—the police—her husband dragged up on a beach breathless—pounding on the chest—failed resuscitations—gawkers—riding in the ambulance to the hospital—accident reports—a funeral. Her life turned upside down.

As images lingered like a scene in a movie, I offered the only words I could, "I'm sorry."

Jackie's eyes welled.

I said, "I never wanted you to go through something like that."

"I almost…lost you." She started crying hard, her chest heaving. I got up from my side of our kitchen booth and sat next to her, holding her. Sat for a long time.

Wiping the tears running down her face, I said, "If it wasn't for you, I wouldn't have made it." She didn't say anything.

A few days after what happened in the waters of Lake Charlevoix, we valiantly tried to put it behind us. We talked about the kids in Chicago and what their plans were for the months ahead. Figuring out a grocery list for the week was a common occurrence in the morning over coffee. We tried to internalize what happened, tried to get back to some kind of normalcy.

Jackie looked as she always did in the morning hours—soft and beautiful. With time buffering what happened the day before, she sipped her black coffee, unlike my cream with some coffee in it. Trying to pull our thoughts to the present, Jackie said, "How about going for a bike ride today? It's great weather, cool, not windy."

Taking all of her in, as I tried to do each morning, I answered, "Only getting up to sixty-two degrees. Not bad, but a bit chilly. Don't know if we want to go all the way up to Harbor Springs or anything."

Jackie always pushed me to get more exercise because she knew my looming coughing and breathing problems were shades of trouble. She also knew that, at sixty-six, I needed to stay in better shape than ever. I tried to balk at working out, but knew she was right. A push was needed.

"Why don't you want to go that far? You go for long bike rides and do well. You said your legs are in good shape after biking all summer."

I answered, "I don't know. Didn't sleep much last night. My coughing kept waking me up."

Jackie didn't say anything and continued eating her veggie omelet. She made really good omelets and always tried to get me to share half. Veggies in the morning—nada. Not even close. Finally, she said, "You know, Zachera has been after you to drive down to Chicago and get a complete physical. With all the coughing and…well…what happened…" She paused, not looking at me. "You need to find out what's going on."

I said, "I know."

I did know, all too well. The impending results of such an exam hovered over me like a dark cloud. Dispelling everything by not going to see a doctor was making it all go away, clearing the clouds. As ignorant as that was, I believed it.

"You need to see Dr. Mike or go see someone in Chicago, like Zachera says."

Whether wanting to say it or believe it, there was only one answer: "I agree."

We finished breakfast. Jackie was right—it was time. Time to face avoidance. It had lasted too long. Time to face the fact that something was really seriously wrong—a roadblock I might not be able to find my way around. My lungs were not ok.

My mother had died from IPF, and Jackie and I were with her throughout her ordeal. Deep inside, I knew I had the same thing. It was exactly why I was resisting tests, appointments, doctors, the whole nine yards. I watched her die. They would find the same thing inside my lungs and I'd be instantly face to face with what my mother went through—her suffering, waking up all night, violent coughing, choking on food, losing her ability to walk, falling in the night, hurting herself, gulping for air as she fumbled for her oxygen mask, and finally turning her oxygen tank up to its highest setting, knowing it was as high as it could go. Knowing she was going to die soon. These were strong, strong images pulling on me, working against my family pleading with me to do something, to move forward, to confront what was happening to my body.

Homeostasis—a state of maintaining normality. We, as humans, have had this state of being inside us for eons. Keep things the same; don't change. There's safety in not changing. Sameness is comforting. Staying where you are feels better to most humans than creating new, challenging scenarios. But we are also aware that sometimes not changing, not moving forward, can lead to our doom—the fragility and impermanence of life on earth.

The older you get, the deeper homeostasis sets in. Ever try to get an older family member to give up driving their car? Difficult. Ever try to get an older person to live in a different place? Almost impossible. We hold on to what we know, what we're used to. We resist.

But it was time to fight the urge to just let things take their course. Jackie and Zachera were right. If I didn't get checked out, the point might come where whatever was wrong couldn't be fixed.

I never imagined what was in front of me.

Paths materialize ahead of you when taking a journey. You may not know exactly where the path is headed and you will definitely come to many crossroads, but when you look back—when your journey's completed—your ride will be memorable—perhaps even extraordinary. We all, at one time or another, experience the road not taken.

Gaining two new donor lungs by way of a double-lung transplant was an incredible journey. Some journeys end. Some keep going in new and different directions. My lung transplant journey hasn't ended. It's part of me and spends daily hours moving around with me in my house, driving into town, sitting quietly while I tell Jackie how much I love her. Two lungs from a donor now residing deep inside me keep me alive. They send precious oxygen to places like Anthony Bourdain's *Parts Unknown*. Hopefully I'll still be around when you're reading these words. We never know.

It's now February 2018, and I'm starting to write about my transplant travels more than two years after my double-lung transplant—a reality never imagined. So, this is what went on, the crazy things that happened, and how it turned out.

People out there who need serious medical attention are about to enter what I call The Twilight Zone. A situation/place in which some of us "human beans" find ourselves. Why? We don't know. In terms of IPF, doctors and scientists at this point don't know either. They're getting closer, but the pieces of the puzzle haven't shown their face. Doctors strive painstakingly to know.

For most of us, the idea of being in a dangerous, life threatening situation doesn't exist. Who goes around on a given day thinking, *Boy, today might be the day I need a new head.* No one. Driving down the expressway, thoughts are on conference championships, fashion, daily news, sales, lunch, cutting the lawn, etc.

The truth is, life threatening things happen to people all the time. Check the national statistics, but be careful when you look them up. Health symptoms on the internet can make you paranoid.

Waking up each day, I move to the side of the bed, sit up on the edge, and take stock. I sit quietly for a moment, like you do, and think about someone else's lungs. Thoughts of my donor family, what happened to them, the courage it took to help, swirl. Do I really do this every single day? Yes. It's not, I surmise, what we all do or think about. A bit different, I understand completely. But concentrating on their kindness is something I do. My lungs will never be taken for granted. Never, ever.

Watching my chest move slightly up and down, I think, *Someone gave me life.* Didn't have to, but they did.

Life is incredibly impermanent—an unmoored boat waiting for a slight breeze. Cat Stevens wrote the song lyrics, "We only dance on this world a short while." Sometimes when we dance, we suspend time and come back. No lesson on metaphysics here, it's just that on my way to dying from an incurable lung disease I received donor lungs and a double-lung transplant. While that was happening, a section of my time on Earth was suspended. Then, I came back.

My transplant journey was extraordinarily intense, one of the biggest moments of my life. Even so, my personal, near death experience seemed only a speck in the integral part of all human experience. One experience in millions and millions of others. We don't exist as a single entity. We're much more connected to each other than we know. The human condition—we're part of everyone.

Sitting next to my father as an eight-year-old at our family's Christmas dinner, my grandfather made a comment I never forgot. He was talking about people in our family who had passed away and how much we missed them. He said, "When a person dies, a library burns down." I wasn't sure why he said it, and, being a young boy, it went right over my head but stuck for some reason. As I got older, I finally realized what it meant.

Each and every one of us has a life story—a book on a library shelf. Our lives are long strings of stories. When we die, our stories, for the most part, stop. Some are remembered for one reason or another, but mostly they, as General MacArthur said, "just fade away."

Our moments exist in a certain realm—a section of time. Einstein's theory of relativity purported the idea that time and space are not constant, that there are sections, blocks, moments of time. I just want you to know so badly that when a family donated their loved one's lungs—when a team of doctors skillfully put them into my body—I was Forrest Gump on his bus-stop bench—suspended.

We don't know everything there is to know, but we do know we're all an important part of everyone else. We are in a connected dimension. We live with time and each other. This thought turned out to be an important and intriguing part of my transplant process. Who would have thought?

Just for me, consider how events definitely move slower or faster depending on what happens within them. Time stops and starts up again. Time warping—Einstein wrote about it years ago. It happened to me. It's happened to you.

How many times have you heard someone describe being in a bad car accident by saying, "Time slowed down, you know? I mean, man, slow motion. I don't know, it was weird. Each exact second...deliberate. Cars moved by me, vehicles that should have been zooming were taking up single spaces, sort of floating. As we were hit, cars swerved back and forth by us like in a movie. I could see their eyes watching me as I watched them."

Time slowing down, halting to rest for a while. Some instances don't always turn out positive. Life gets its balance. But they're snapshots of time: a police officer pulling a woman from a burning car, a jogger saving a drowning child from a river, a train hitting a bus. Moments interconnected.

Sitting with my mother beside her bed when she died was one.

Seconds that take a hundred times longer than they should. Mom and I in her small bedroom. Just the two of us. An incredible, beautiful woman knew she was dying. She talked to me a week before and asked if I'd promise to come over—by myself—the following Wednesday night. I promised. The look on her face was both intense and wanting. It was no ordinary request.

That Wednesday, we spent the evening together. She was in her bed and I was in a chair next to her. We held hands for quite a while and said we loved each other. She fell gently asleep. I sat still for a while, not wanting to wake her. Our small town sounds an old-fashioned ten thirty curfew siren every evening. Mom stopped breathing seconds before the siren went off. Now, years later, if the wind is right at our house, we can faintly hear our town's ten thirty siren wafting through the trees. I always stop and listen.

When my daughter Zachera was born, she wasn't breathing. The doctor whisked our baby to a steel table ten feet away while I stood next to Jackie's hospital bed. Jackie couldn't tell what was going on and kept looking up at me with wonder in her eyes. Something wasn't right. All I could see was the doctor's back and his arms moving up and down, intent nurses on each side. Time stopped. Suddenly, a shrill cry, and then another and another. Zachera entered our world. As nurses wrapped her up in a blanket to take to Jackie, the doctor turned. "She's going to be alright. Her lung was collapsed, but we were able to help her, and she's breathing just fine." He turned and walked out of the room to go help another patient. Just like that. Incredible work. Life.

Jackie gazed at the child she had just brought into the world. Amazement and joy. All of this took six or seven minutes, but it hadn't. It had taken a lifetime. Some days just hang out in the median. Others are extraordinary sparks that keep us constantly in awe.

3

Snapshots

There were lots of sparks in the early sixties. We were kids born this or that side of 1950. But there was a specific set of days that made an indelible impression on everyone living in the United States at the time, and for years to come.

It's important to describe these three days because they are perfect examples of life in suspended sections…all interconnected. They represent how fragile we are, how we're only here for one fleeting moment in time. My donor family deciding to give me their loved one's organs. The masterful surgeon painstakingly placing two lungs in my open chest.

November 1963. We all hung out for an adjourned set of days… but not because we wanted to. Ask anyone who went through it. Do they remember? Absolutely, because they were there…and then they were back. The musical *Rocky Horror Picture Show* has a dance number describing it: "Doin' the Time Warp."

A closer look at this particular circumstance will help. For those born after 1960, you were three years old or younger, or didn't exist yet. You may only know about this event from books, movies, television documentaries, panel discussions, and conspiracy theories.

If you lived through those three days, they've become a still life painting. Each and every minute stands out like describing that car accident. Time became far from ordinary.

I was a young boy of thirteen sitting in front of our black-and-white

Zenith TV set. Shows back then consisted of *Lassie, The Lone Ranger, The Howdy Doody Show,* and other boring programs our parents watched, like *Lawrence Welk* or *The Ed Sullivan Show.* Well, ok, Ed Sullivan did have Topo Gijo, a funny mouse, but the rest were yawners to a seventh grader: old-guy singers with slicked-back hair, a guy juggling plates on a stick, and women with weird platinum hair.

But there was one show that mesmerized us kids. Some parents wouldn't let their kids watch it. Too scary. *The Twilight Zone* was the perfect metaphor for suspended time. Rod Sterling, in his dark suit, would walk onto the screen with large, menacing black eyebrows, dark inset eyes and say: "You're traveling through another dimension, a dimension not only of sight and sound…but of mind. That signpost up ahead—your next stop—The Twilight Zone!"

I had to watch. We all did. Eerie things were happening.

November 22, 1963

On a particularly gray late-fall Friday, my friends and I were in elementary school—Hampton Elementary School—in northwest Detroit. They call it middle school now, but back then K-8 was simply called elementary school.

My best friend Charlie and I were in Mr. Doud's science classroom, sitting in old wooden chairs with small, cutting-board-like platforms to swing up and write on. My chair's wooden platform had "yor butt" carved into it.

Mr. Doud was a thin, older teacher with graying hair he was trying to color. He stood about six feet two. Kids called him Ichabod. He'd drone on and on trying to get us interested in science. To liven up class, he'd pass out *Science Magazine*, which was a cheap publication for elementary students. It was free to all of us, so you can imagine.

Science Magazine was only three pieces of pulpy paper folded in half, but it had a section called "The Future!" We couldn't wait to read "The Future!" because it revealed new and cool stuff. I mean, it was the future, come on. It talked about crazy stuff like in comic books, but for real! It referred to "the cutting sword" or "edge" or something. There were articles about how cars were going to be "hovercrafts" zoomin' around with no wheels! Goin' anywhere you wanted in any direction, even up and down! The problem is, I've been waiting sixty-eight years—hasn't happened. Kind of like the Detroit Lions.

While deeply entrenched in "The Future!" all of a sudden, the upper corner classroom speaker sounded off: "Bong...Bong.... Bong...Children, this is your principal speaking. An awful thing has happened, but don't be scared. President Kennedy has been shot in Dallas, Texas. Please stay seated. School will be let out when Mrs. Winslout announces your classroom. Buses will be lined up in the front of the school as usual. For those of you walking home, please go straight home to your mothers. If you need a ride home, please come to the front office and we will let you use our phone or drive you home. Thank you."

Everyone in the classroom was in shock. Some girls started screaming. Mr. Doud told everyone to stay seated and be quiet. Be quiet?! President John F. Kennedy had been shot and killed. Everything was crazy. All the teachers were in a state of panic. Later on that day, news broadcasts would run clips of Walter Cronkite taking off his glasses, looking solemnly into the camera, and, in a deep voice, explaining our president was dead. It ran over and over on the TV.

In those days, most kids had a mother at home during the day. My mom was way ahead of her time. She had a full-time job, made more money than my dad, and had her own sports car. She was very hip. I was allowed to be home by myself. And, no, nothing bad ever happened to me because of it.

School let out around one thirty. I was surprised at how upset and sad everyone was. Teachers were ignoring our normal pushing and shoving and were talking to each other in deep tones. One teacher—who had black hair and gorgeous eyes, and whom I had a major crush on—ran out to her car and drove frantically out of the teachers' parking lot.

On my walk home, people were out on their front porches, talking and waving their arms. I mean, it was terrible. People loved President Kennedy. They respected politicians back then. Once home, my best friend, Charlie, sped into my backyard on his bike and jumped off, letting it crash into our garage. We all did that.

Charging through our kitchen door, Charlie yelled, "Hey, mambo jambo! School's out! Kinda weird." He lived two houses down and loved to bear hug you until you said, "I give!" He was a big guy with a round, red-cheeked face. Our neighborhood in Detroit had large families and was mainly Catholic, which explained it. A lot of Jewish people lived on the other side of Seven Mile in the bigger, more expensive homes.

Once out of Charlie's Sasquatch grip, I caught my breath and said, "Gotta love it, school's out, but...yeah...this assassination thing, huh?"

"They got the one who shot 'em. Crazy nuts!"

"You said it, jeeeeshish!" I handed Charlie a cold milk bottle for a swig.

After the third gulp, Charlie swiped his sleeve and said, "My mom was crying when I got home."

"What?! No kiddin'?"

"No kiddin'. It was scary. I thought Aunt Phillis finally died or somethin'. She's like three hundred years old. Mom just kept crying."

"Your mom is always cheery. I've never seen her cry or stuff like that."

"I know." Charlie added, "It's this President Kennedy thing. She thought he was the greatest, always talking about him and some Camelot stuff..."

"I don't know. Pretty strange," I said.

Our country was in a complete flux and all our neighbors were talking about Russians comin'. Who did it? Speculations flew. Khrushchev and the Communists? Fidel Castro? Was it that Bay of Pigs thing in Cuba? Some said they captured a "lone shooter" named Os—somewhere in downtown Dallas. A movie theatre.

Others said it was more than one man and they were behind a grassy knoll, whatever the hell that is?

There were a lot of bulletins and special reports on TV. My mom made me skip mass on Sunday—which neverrrr happens—because I had a nasty sore throat. Normally, on Sunday after mass, I'd be playing street hockey with the guys. But Mom put her foot down. "Robert, if you are too sick to miss mass, you're too sick to be outside. Besides when a child gets cold, they get a cold!" Common myth back then, but there was no tellin' Mom that.

Dad and Mom were heading out that afternoon to Birmingham, a suburb of Detroit, for something called a "Chip and Dip" party. They were going to leave me home alone, as usual. In those days kids could stay home alone. I'm not sure what changed?

Dad said, "Listen to your mother. She's told you to stay inside and that's what you'll do, right?" Strict instructions I'd have to follow. Neighbors watched us like hawks and if I was out playing hockey with my buddies, my parents would know about it before I did.

"Got homework and stuff, Dad, so I'll stay inside. Don't worry."

"Oh…and take the trash out. Tomorrow's trash day," he added, heading out the door.

Parents always said things like that. If I couldn't go outside to play hockey, how come I could take the trash out?

As my parents backed down our narrow driveway in Dad's blue Chevrolet Bellaire and headed north, kids in the street yelled, "Carrrr!" and moved to the curb with their hockey sticks and net. It's what you did.

Looking out our living-room window at my friend's street hockey game made me feel crappy, so I plopped on the sofa and started doing absolutely nothing, which is what you do when your parents go out. Homework could wait until whenever. Actually, I wasn't being completely useless—I was peeling a tangerine so the peel didn't break and carefully putting it back together to fool Dad. He always acted like it was a whole one. When I got older, I realized Dad and Mom made like a lot of things were true that really weren't to build up my confidence. Totally worked.

I turned our TV's flimsy plastic knob (remotes didn't exist) and saw an ad for Jiffy Pop, which didn't sound half bad. Of course, we didn't have any. The Detroit Lions would be on later, but they hadn't won a game since Columbus and 1492. Noon TV on Sunday was not a hotbed of entertainment. In fact, it was awful. There was always an old white-haired guy with lots of wrinkles reading a Bible with a purple-haired lady with smeared red lipstick smiling next to him. She would look down to play an organ and then look back up and smile like she just farted.

We only had NBC, ABC, and CBS then. That was it...three channels. If you're younger, you laugh at only three channels. And, yes, there were telephone booths—Angry Birds only existed on lawns—text meant words in a book—and Spotify was carpet cleaner. Different time, different place.

We did, however, get Canadian channel 9 since Windsor, Canada was just across the Detroit River. Channel 9 was Canada's hockey channel, and, come NHL playoff time, we watched Gordie Howe and the Detroit Red Wings faithfully.

Dad and I never missed a Wings playoff game. Nothing was more exciting than to watch the seventh game of the Stanley Cup Finals: third period, down two to one against the Montreal Canadiens—Wings pull goalie Terry Sawchuk—one minute to go!—Delvecchio shoots—clang!—the announcer screams, "He hit the post—Ted Lindsay clobbers their defenseman in front of the net—Gordie swoops in behind for the rebound!" The announcer goes wild, "Howe shoots! He scores!! Gordie Howe scores!! It's two to two! The game is tied!!" We would jump up and run around the room with our arms raised! When Dad got quite old and in poor health, I'd come over to be with him and if the Wings scored, he couldn't get up, but he'd still raise his arms up in the air with me.

So, there I was on a Sunday with senseless Sunday TV. I got up and turned the dial—click—a wrestling show. Mom wouldn't let me watch Big Time Wrestling because she said it was fake. I was insanely bored. My boredom didn't last long.

Suddenly, NBC cut in with a special report:...didit...didit...didit...

didit. A large red screen took up the whole TV. It had the words "NEWS BULLETIN" written boldly in the middle. "We will now go to a live broadcast of Lee Harvey Oswald being taken from the downtown Dallas jailhouse." Who was this guy?!

Whatever this interruption was, it had to be part of all the hullaba-loo from President Kennedy being shot on Friday when we were in school. The announcer was speaking in an overly concerned voice, like each word he was saying was going to go down in history or something. He whispered, "We are here, live, in Dallas, Texas."

I thought to myself, *No kidding. What would you be…dead there in Dallas?* The guy continued, "We're hearing lots of noise now…talk…Just a minute…we're being told Dallas police will be bring-ing Oswald out momentarily. It might be a…wait…I see some-thing going on up by what appears to be an exit door…Yes…they seem to be bringing Oswald out. He has handcuffs on. Two large officers have ahold of Oswald on each side through his arms. A car has pulled up by the alley entrance, presumably for Oswald's transport."

Cameras were trained on the alley and there were bright, large flood lights on. Suddenly, as the cops pulled Oswald through the crowd, this old guy with a hat stepped out from the side of the crowd with what looked like a pistol. The two large cops appeared to be holding Oswald open, like a target, and then the man in the hat shot Oswald in the chest. The announcer screamed, "Oswald's been shot! Oswald's been shot!" I kept eating my tangerine. People on the screen were yelling and screaming. Police officers jumped on Oswald and the old guy. It was chaos.

Cameras and lights were being jostled around and one fell over. The live TV feed went blank and the screen switched to a news guy at a desk.

I just sat there, at thirteen years old, trying to take in what I had just witnessed. My parents weren't home—no one was around to talk to—I couldn't go out. John F. Kennedy was gone forever. I watched a man named Ruby shoot another man named Oswald live on television...My tangerine was supposed to help my sore throat.

Jackie and I were sitting in a Chicago doctor's office listening to my pulmonary specialist tell us I needed a lung transplant to keep from dying. IPF had no cure, he said. No cure. Just as those three days in 1963 existed outside of my normal life—so did almost getting killed by gang members on a downtown Detroit truck dock—so did 9/11. Just separate shelves.

But the days surrounding my lung transplant existed in a different way. Hours didn't last days, a weekend didn't last a month, as did other halted moments. This time, it was further away...off on its own. I'll never know, but maybe it was the transplant—different human beings becoming, somehow, one.

On a cold November day in 2015, Jackie and I left our home in northern Michigan and drove down our tree-lined driveway to Chicago to see if there was something doctors could do to save me.

3 1/2

Side Note

I know, I know...there's no such thing as half-chapters! Sorry, it's necessary. Won't take long...promise.

First, if you've read this far, you know names have been changed on purpose, including my hospital's name, MMHMMM—Mercy Mercy Hospital Mother Mary Mercy. This mouthful came from a conglomeration of crazy hospital names I've witnessed: Lady Fatima of the Slightly Bottomless; Mother Jones Hospital for Scamming; The Sick Place (I'm not going there); and Willy's Pretty Good Hospital for Dolls and Humans.

By the way, how come 90 percent of hospitals use female nomenclature? Think Mary Queen of Scots Quick Head Care, or Wonder Women's Hospital for the Seriously Squeezed. Ok, women are the nurturing ones, I get that, but guys never, ever take care of anyone? No guys? Evidently guys only mess with cars and football, then die? That's it. How about hospitals with guy names? Mac's Fix-a-Dick or Pa's Clinic for the Flatulent? I know they use Father in some hospital titles, but it's rare. When I was in Colorado, there was a FFRMHMH—Father Flinn's Rocky Mountain High Mountain Hospital—which was probably a nod to John Denver and Colorado's recent law changes. I don't know.

Second, I really did get a double-lung transplant. This book isn't fiction. If you meet me someday, I'll show you my cool scars. They're great at parties.

Third, if you must have stuff done in a hospital, figure out hospital lingo ASAP. Not understand it, mind you, just recognize it when it comes whizzing by.

When you zing through the hospital's revolving doors, you enter a bizarre world. No kidding. Just figuring out how to get a parking voucher, let alone paying for one, will entail an educated, intrinsic understanding of a crazy and zany world called your medical center.

With your rectangular parking ticket firmly in hand, the information-desk person will say, "That ticket be the one you put in the parking slot when you leave, honey. Find the white box thang wid a slot. Where's your blue slip with green stripes that says lot 50K132? Ahhhh, ok, that the one you want punched, not this Macy's receipt." So, it's what you think you know vs. the hospital's strategy to make sure you don't know.

Without creating too much angst here, prepare to enter a fun hospital acronym world tour. Everything will be labeled by first letters. Because you have no prior knowledge of this letter / word / canned ham / Wally World deal, everything will soon morph into crazy shit that just happens. I hate to call it that, but your check-in papers and pamphlets are proof.

Why a half-chapter? Because you probably don't like surprises. Some people love being scared shitless by surprises. On Halloween these people go to haunted houses and have someone jump on them or put gooey things in their hair. They actually pay money to do this. They run through some local fire station screaming bloody murder with their hands above their head. Then, after it's over and they get dry underwear, they laugh their asses off.

It's the spider thing. I hate spiders. Not so much because of the way they look or crawl—ok, partly—but because the damn things surprise you! If they'd just tap you on the shoulder and say, "Hey, excuse me, but I'm on your collar...no biggie." Butttt they don't! Eight legs—what's with that, anyway? I'm just eliminating surprises.

Don't let hospital acronyms, urine-colored masks, cold x-ray plates, bedpans, rubber Jell-O, abandoned gurneys with patients in them, or slippery shit surprise you. Be prepared! Read the pamphlets! They won't make sense, but read them. It will show you're willing to try. Some people get so overwhelmed going in they say, "Nope," walk back to their car, and go home. This is actually legal. You can do this. Your doctors didn't want me to tell you, but I felt obligated.

There you go. Thanks for participating.

4

Someone Else's Lungs

Stories are who we were when—and who we are today. After completing my lung transplant initial recovery and being back home resting in our living room looking out at a small section of forest, I took stock. General health was good, no coughing, food was starting to taste semi-normal. It just felt bizarre sitting there... with someone else's lungs in my body.

During that quiet moment, a song ran through my head over and over—Paul McCartney's "Maybe I'm Amazed." I was...truly. It was the thought that summed up everything that happened to me. Amazed. Amazed at the strength of my family, at their unending support, amazed at my friends who visited me in Chicago when I was badly off, at MMHMMM's staff and how they took care of me at every single turn. There were lots and lots of turns and at each one—I was amazed.

Life had moved on in our little woods. The fox family living under the downed trees from a winter storm would visit our backyard that evening on their way to the lake for water. Squirrels would dance their way around every which way, making no sense. The deer had eaten some of Jackie's perennial garden, but we expected their visit since no one had been home. They had free range.

Jackie had headed into town for groceries. Sitting there quietly—northern Michigan quiet—I heard it—the silence. When Zachera and Ryan visit from where they live in downtown Chicago, they have trouble sleeping the first night. They say, "It's just too damn quiet here!" From the second night on, they sleep like children.

But the silence raised a question: How did all this happen? Why? How did I end up with one of the top lung transplant surgeons in the country? How did donor lungs come to me and make "a perfect fit," as my surgeons said? How did my body make it through being almost cut in half to get my old lungs out and new lungs in? Where did my blood go? How did my heart keep beating? It was the same body that got thrashed around on a rugby field, the same body that hadn't been taken perfect care of through the years. Why was I still sitting here after a ravaging, life ending disease attacked my lungs? No answer. Will there ever be one? Not sure. Silence.

Here's what happened. What a simple sentence, all things considered. A double-lung transplant procedure has a scope far bigger than most know. In fact, most don't know it exists. Many people said to me, "A double-lung transplant? Didn't know they could do that." Taking part in one was an enormous event. Turned out, it ended up being a whole lot of events strung together. To tell you about every one of them would be too many. Some too grim to write about. Also, there were times I wasn't coherent enough—the meds—to know where my toes were. "Excuse me, Lowinda," I said to my nurse, "I don't know...but yesterday...ahhhh...I had toes. They don't seem to be down there?"

Lowinda's answers always put a smile on my face: "Y'all got toes, sugarrrr. Believe me when I say!"

I do remember some parts, though. Many are significant because of the humans who made them possible: doctors, nurses, staff. My transplant was not only vast, but, in some ways, even bigger for my family. Physically large for me, yes, but they had to weather my surgery along with what was going to happen if I didn't make it. Thoughts in that vein are inconceivable, overwhelming. I don't even want to go there. For me, enduring tough moments alive wasn't even close to dealing with death. One is fighting to live; the other is over. Days move on; death is final.

Taken all in all, my journey wouldn't have even started if it hadn't been for Jackie. Jackie has been by my side just about all my life. We were high-school sweethearts, married after both receiving degrees from Michigan State University (MSU), and, with teaching certificates in hand, we headed to the northern Michigan woods to make educational history. I smile at the thought.

Jackie helps me, loves me. Always will to "the third star on the right, and straight on 'til morning." In terms of my lungs, Jackie was the person who first noticed symptoms of pulmonary fibrosis, got me to stop being stubborn and go see a doctor. She stood by me through all the initial tests. Jackie and Zachera were the ones who insisted on visiting a newly formed lung transplant team in Chicago. They made it happen. Yes, there were brief discussions with a pulmonary specialist in Petoskey, Michigan, but either there were no appointments for months or my appointment was cancelled when I showed up. True story. All roads led to Chicago, with luck along for the ride.

As it turned out, there were five people who initially set things in motion: Jackie; my incredible daughter Zachera, who vehemently insisted on MMHMMM; Ryan, who set up everything with Zachera in Chicago; my close friend and hometown primary doctor; and a sweet, dear friend named Julie who worked at MMHMMM. Had it not been for these five special people, these lines would be white on white.

MMHMMM built a transplant dream team just over a year before I arrived. They put together top surgeons from around the world to form one of the most esteemed transplant teams in the U.S. And I was in the middle of it all.

Lucky, again and again. It was a new program with impeccable reviews. American Medical Association journal articles were written about it. So it was that Jackie, Zachera, and Ryan were in my hand and heart as I was wheeled through the surgery doors to survive a ten-hour double-lung transplant—to fight for a chance to breathe again.

My journey went from denial, to lung specialist, to tedious testing, to a transplant. Jackie, Zachera, and Ryan were next to me while in surgery, post-surgical recovery, physical therapy, getting me out of bed, standing next to me putting my feet on the floor for the first time, ambling slowly down the long halls of the seventh floor as I slowly gained strength. How lucky I was to have them hold my arms sitting down on a handy dandy shower chair, making me—willing or not—do my exercises, or urge me to take one more step up in the hospital stairway.

Zachera visited me as much as she could, took vital time out of her working day, spent evenings having strange crockpot dinners in our little hotel room across from the hospital. She continually got me to do the right thing medically. Jackie, Zachera, and Ryan got me here today, looking out at a beautiful forest with one thought repeating like a ticker tape, *If it wasn't for Jackie, Zachera, and Ryan*...over and over.

Just so you know, as you read along, this isn't a thriller where I capture a criminal, surprise the hell out of you at every turn, save my roommate—who later becomes the most interesting person in the world—or use the Heimlich maneuver on a choking woman in Greektown who turns out to be Nancy Reagan. Nothing terrible happened to me in terms of a Code Red, unless maybe they didn't tell me? Well, ok, there were moments, but I'm telling you up front there were no aliens bursting out of my chest, no superhuman feats of dragging myself up seventeen flights of stairs to the ICU only to find they were closed for cleaning. I don't want you jumping sky high from fright or waiting for an exciting part on pins and needles. (Who waits "on pins and needles"? What the hell issss that?) You already know I made it through because of the title and because, "Hi, how you doing?" No suspense. This is more about people and moments.

My double-lung transplant went incredibly well—I have to just straight out tell you. How that happened is another matter and fills these pages. I was wheeled out the same operating room doors I went in. Actually, those doors became quite metaphorical. I still get emotional thinking about them. Doors swinging into possibly the end of my life—doors swinging back out—alive.

After my ten-hour operation, the orderly pushing my gurney hit the big metal "open" button and those entry/exit doors swung apart. Out I came—a living person. It was a lot like being born, but I'm not going there. Being driven along on the gurney, I didn't know a thing. It was a meadow called Never Never Land, but the doctors knew. Coming out those doors was ethereal—a moment close to my heart.

The surgery was dangerous. My doctors said it was fifty-fifty at best. But, here's the thing: incredible human beings saved me. Here and there in my now new daily life, people ask me, "How in the world did you do it?" Then I start to think, *How did I?* Taken all in all, it was simply time to get in the batter's box. During surgery, I was just there, period—no wondering, chatting, cellphone, singing, or playing board games. It was all a tale full of magnificent human beings, modern medicine and science, on all possible levels.

Some of the patients' stories surrounding me, next to me, in rooms down the hall from me at MMHMMM's lung transplant center didn't end up positive. Some patients took months and months to heal and have their lungs work properly. Some of their stories ended. When we die, our stories become Kansas's "dust in the wind." Reality. Why did things go so well for me, but not so well for others? Lots of factors I suppose, but...I really don't know.

I was slowly dying. Each day, my lungs transferred less oxygen. If you would, please, stop for a moment and take a long, deep breath and hold it...(I know, but just for me, ok?)...Feel what it's like...When your oxygen level starts to drop, you can feel it and you start to get anxious. When you can't hold your breath any more, it gets intense. You let out a burst and take in all the air you can.

For patients with malfunctioning lungs, what you just experienced can be, in some ways, part of their day. If these patients start coughing, it can become a frightening struggle waiting for air to fill your lungs once again. As my IPF lung disease got worse, when taking a breath, it felt like nothing went in. They still felt empty. Sometimes it felt like I couldn't take a breath at all, like my lungs had stopped working altogether. You might have viewed movie scenes like in *Titanic*, where someone is trapped and water is starting to come up and over their head. They're gulping for air, but running out of space. Breathing becomes panic.

Levels of panic would come and go. Sometimes those feelings would subside, but you never knew when they were going to occur. That was the worst part. It didn't happen often, but worrying about it wore on you. Maybe it would happen when out with friends at a restaurant, maybe at a movie. You started to second guess doing things, went out less often for fear it would happen.

Soon, I couldn't exist without my oxygen tank. My life was slipping. I started on "Level Two." The dial went from one to five. Looking at my tank's dial was ominous—every time. Ominous because if I was on a two, at some point it would be a five. Five is your life's visible numerical limit. Your outlook takes on a much different hue. At first, I tried to keep from changing the number. I'd try to stay on two, but no matter how I tried, my lungs would start to ask for more of the oxygen I took for granted all my life. Then three, then four. One morning, when I turned my tank to five because I couldn't breathe, it finally hit me. That was it. I couldn't turn it up anymore. That morning I started to cry. My life was going to end soon.

But then, near what would have been the end, I was given a gift by a loving couple. A gift like no other gift. A couple who, during a time of intense personal grief, donated their loved one's lungs to me. To me. Writing this still brings up a welling in my heart.

To grasp completely why I'm breathing and living today is going to take time—a long time. Time to understand, to put in perspective. I'm not sure I ever will. It's far bigger than me, bigger than anything I've experienced when viewed in terms of what it really is. I'm still trying to get my head around that.

Looking at death firsthand is beyond scary because it's the unknown. Doubts creep into your mind constantly. *Should I go ahead with this surgery? Maybe it would be better to just let things go? My family is going to have to go through too much. I don't want to be a burden, and I could certainly end up one. I want my family's lives to be happy, not spent taking care of me, trying to hold my head up, trying to help me live on when maybe I shouldn't.*

Maybe thoughts and details here will help patients be less scared. The unknown is far better facing forward with knowledge. I lived, and now ride my bike through the woods every day or snowshoe in the winter. Knowing what other survivors know would have helped while contemplating a transplant. I wish someone had called me when I was depressed and said, "Hey, I'm living. I had what you have. I got new lungs. I'm alive. I'm ok! You'll be ok, too."

The fact that patients die is all too real. Speaking to someone who survived could have helped because dying was so imminent. No need to dwell on statistics—what's needed is hope. A clear light. A "go" indicating it all might work. Listening to doctors is somehow different. You know they're going to say everything will be fine. I hesitate to call it "the company line," because that sounds so crass, but that's what it is. They have to say the correct thing and it's important they do. But let's be honest, doctors can't spend time going over all the mental aspects of your situation like a former patient can. Patients want personal insight into where they're headed, reality from someone who has been there. They want to know what they are in for—in real time—so they can prepare to battle mightily and come back—keep on keeping on. Every patient knows they might die. What they want is a positive ray of light.

In my life, I've always handled things better with knowledge of the task. It's kind of like the "tools needed for the job" list that comes with a DIY product. Knowledge. Dealing with the unknown is much more difficult. Knowing, you can make a plan, buck up, do whatever it takes to be ready. I had no idea whatsoever what was going to happen once my lungs stopped functioning, and once my whole ordeal started.

After meeting and talking to patients entering into the lung transplant process, the most notable thing that stood out above all else was their fear. Talking to one couple who were waiting to be put on the national donor list, the husband started trembling. He had the same feelings as the man in the wheelchair I spoke of earlier. That it was all "too much," too overwhelming, no control. He was terrified. It was then that I knew details, format, schedules, doctors, procedures, days in the hospital, all of it—any of it—could help. Knowing where you're headed beats being lost.

Some might think knowing these things early might scare a patient, make them uncertain. This was a concern and I always asked them after Paul set up our meeting if they wanted to talk or not. It was ok if they didn't. But each and every patient wanted to know everything, all of it, ahead of time.

Meeting a lung transplant team and talking to a lung surgeon certainly is the first step in facing this unknown. Dr. Danzor, my pulmonary doctor, told me transplanting lungs from one human being to another is the largest surgery in medicine. The enormity of his statement didn't hit me until one late night, when Zachera, Jackie, and I were quietly discussing what was about to take place. We were in our hotel room across the street from MMHMMM. I had to be in close proximity to the hospital when and if the team called to say they had donor lungs that were a good fit.

I was sitting in a lounge chair facing the TV. Jackie and Zachera were sitting on a brown, weathered, nondescript couch against the wall. The TV was on, but the sound was turned off. The hotel refrigerator had a weird hum. MMHMMM's team was deciding the next day whether they would place me on the national transplant list or not. Was it the right time? Did I qualify? Had they covered every detail? Could I survive the ordeal? Should I do this? Should I stop? We knew it was going to be touchy. I was sixty-six years old. Seventy was the cutoff. They had to save viable lungs for patients who were young enough, strong enough, and well enough to go through the transplant and live. It made sense. Life was for the living.

In the midst of our quiet conversation that night, it hit me. All of it, all at once. Everything the doctors were saying, everything they were describing, the ramifications, everyone involved, the magnitude. I broke down. It all rushed in on me. All I remember was saying, blurry-eyed, "It's all too big, you know. Really large. The operation is the biggest there is. It's way big…I don't know… maybe it's too much." A waterfall of emotions poured out. I had been holding them inside, trying to be strong, trying to make it so my family wouldn't have to go through it, trying to make it no big deal, working on every end run I could to somehow get out of it. But it was there—standing in front of me—it could be tomorrow. It was happening, and I couldn't hold it back any longer.

A double-lung transplant is extreme and complicated. Going through with it was going to affect many people I loved. There was a fifty-fifty chance of not making it through surgery. I might die. What was Jackie going to do? How would Zachera, my only child, deal with it? Thoughts blew up in my brain. We couldn't afford it, couldn't waste our whole life savings. What if I came out alive but things didn't go well? What if Jackie had to coddle me for years; what if I couldn't talk or walk afterwards?

Breaking down so severely wasn't something I wanted to do in front of my daughter. Jackie and I had been through a lot together and we'd done our share of crying and letting emotions overtake us for good reasons, but we always handled it. I was worried Zachera would get scared along with me. That was the last thing I wanted. I didn't want anyone to be affected. I could take the heat, the brunt of it. I could be strong and had been tough in my life, but a decision to go ahead with this could ruin too many things for Zachera, Jackie, and the rest of our family. Maybe I shouldn't go through with it? Maybe I should keep going along the same way. I could last for a while. My head just kept blaring, *You might die if you do this. You might die.*

There in our small room that night, I couldn't stop the deep rush of emotions inside me from erupting. I cried even harder. My hidden thoughts came pouring out. My chest was heaving. All I remember saying was, "This is big. This is so f——ing big. Just so damn huge, guys. All of this…I can't imagine any of this, all of this." It was true, I couldn't. But inside I knew it had to happen. The alternative lurked in front of me, a dark animal with deliberate eyes. If I didn't try, I'd eventually lose my ability to breathe and die. I'd watched my mother die the same way. Did I want to leave my family? Did I want to see the end of my time? No. It was a massive emotional crash.

Jackie and Zachera calmed me down. They talked me through my deep-felt concerns. It ended up being extremely good because I let it out. Jackie kept saying, "We'll make it. We'll be alright." She didn't know that any more than I did, but the thing was... she totally believed it, 100 percent. And, here's the thing, Jackie never—ever—stopped being completely positive. She said, "We'll get through this, and then we'll be back home. The team knows what they're doing, and they're the best there is. You don't have to worry about the money. Insurance will help. Money shouldn't be any part of this. I know this is huge, but it is what it is and your job is to be strong and get through it. You can. You've always been strong."

Throughout the whole ordeal, Jackie continued to be positive, no matter what. On the other hand, what was happening to me started to become too much for Zachera. She was just twenty-five and had never had a family member die, at least when she was old enough to understand. She was only four when my parents died. Zachera's other grandparents were still going strong in their nineties. It wasn't until Zachera was in college that she faced the death of our twelve-year-old dog, Holly. But she wasn't there. There's something about being there, something exceedingly real.

How would Zachera do with all this? She had just gotten married to a fine gentleman named Ryan. How would this affect their relationship? She had worked incredibly hard to start her own photography company and was swamped with work. How would her career be affected?

Zachera stayed strong even though she was frightened. She tried to help, to be with me, to do whatever she could. When we'd sit together, she'd talk about what I taught her. Things like, "Life is all about getting in the batter's box." She said, "When I messed up or things didn't go well, when I was depressed, you used to ask me your proverbial question, 'Why do we fall down?' If I didn't remember, you'd always remind me, 'To learn how to get back up.'" Looking at me deeply, Zachera said, "Dad, it's your turn now."

Zachera was right. It was my turn. If you're going lay out platitudes, you needed to stand by them. After my emotional Netflix, episode six, chapter three-type incident, I tried to breathe slowly. Jackie brought me a towel. I was a mess. It was that night with two of the people I love the most my odyssey became oddly simple. It was as if the fog cleared on a lonely highway. All those negative thoughts stopped. It was now one single thought: *Time to get up. I must do this. So what if it's enormous, so what if it's going to be painful, so what if recovery is long? It's simple—it's what I'm going to do.* And…that was it.

I slept well that night. What was so strange about that prior evening was I never looked back. Not once. There was never a period of doubt after that night with Jackie and Zachera. That night needed to happen and eventually was going to happen. It was then that I set myself to the task—arrived at my intention. It was happening and I was going to make it. My compass was set that special evening. My whole experience was set on "go."

I had come to the conclusion that whatever happened when I came out of those surgery room doors was what was going to happen. I'd fight with everything I had to make it work because it was what I wanted. It was what Zachera and Jackie wanted me to do, needed me to do. Deep down inside—and I mean at the base of my base—I felt an incredibly strong urge to keep going—not to quit on myself, Jackie, Zachera, Ryan, or anyone. I didn't conjure it up—it just arrived. Plain and simple.

Later, people would ask me, "How did you do it? How did you get through all that?" Those questions always set me back a bit because for me it was a mindset; it was simple. To others it probably didn't make sense.

Simple? They wanted a much more complicated explanation. To them, it had to be more. Of course, it was complicated. But, for me, my intent—my resolve—dawned like a sunrise.

5

Not an Epilogue

What saved my life after contracting IPF came in one enormous wave and then in specific pieces. That's the way life seems to go—pieces of the puzzle. Big parts, then smaller parts. A major part—a loving organ donor who was in the midst of extreme grief summoned up the courage to donate to the national organ donor organization. Because of what she did when her husband died—a decision made somewhere miles and miles away—I am now breathing on my own again. There's no way I can put into words what this woman did for me. I now walk out into a cold, snowy morning and visually watch my breath. It forms before me like tiny dandelion seeds wafting in the wind.

Every single day I feel this special family's donation in my body. My lungs move up and down, side to side. They work away doing their important job—they keep me alive. My donor lungs represent an act of pure and simple love from another human being. I want to let my donor family out there know what a difference they have made in another person's life, in another family's life. There's no other way to put it: I thank them from the bottom of my heart.

My donor and I have communicated anonymously. We don't know names, hospitals, or any information leading to a breach of privacy. Our anonymous letters are taken care of by the national donor association, so neither of us has to feel pressured or guilty. I will always love someone I don't even know.

These words are necessary because I couldn't possibly start writing about what transpired daily down the transplant road without first telling you about the person who made it happen.

There was a surprise waiting for me when I started writing this book. From the very first page, it became clear the experience was going to be cathartic. Fine, I'll come clean, I kept a towel sitting next to my keyboard. While writing, emotions come streaming out, sentiments I didn't see coming, or expected from deep inside. They harken back to feelings in the hospital room, in surgery, being in the ICU, gliding down a long hallway on a gurney, seeing people look as we wheeled by. Overwhelming feelings I buried deep inside or hadn't worked through yet. They became real, raw, and vividly clear once I touched them.

Paul, my clinical psychologist, probably urged me to write because he knew it would help. He's pretty damn smart, so I wouldn't put it past him. He knew going back and reliving everything that would waken inner thoughts, open up a vessel full of suppressed emotions. He also knew it would heal me in many ways during my stay at MMHMMM and afterward. I owe him—he spends his days helping people. He's a good person. It's not a job to him, it's a vocation.

Mild symptoms of post-traumatic stress disorder (PTSD) have cropped up since my surgery. It's nothing close to the PTSD some people have from awful, awful experiences—not that serious, but it's there. Sometimes, out of the blue, flashes of situations, operating rooms, patients, and doctors appear and send my mind whirling. I never know when they're going to hit me. They never last long, but they throw me, they take me back. Paul knew. One day Jackie asked from the kitchen why I closed our den door when writing. I told her, in my best Al Pacino impression, "Becausssse...I'm self-conscious...I'm gettin' emotional heeeere." Every chapter brought this on, I can tell you.

None of us really know what lies in the depths of our mind until something's triggered. Sometimes feelings erupt like a volcano. Occasionally they come quietly like a cool breeze. One morning while writing, I started to cry. Didn't know what was happening or why. Couldn't stop. Memories came crashing in. I finally got up and went for a long walk in the woods. When I came back, I felt really good, like something lifted.

How much do we internalize? Certainly, it's a lot more than we outwardly know. So, on one February day when a family donated a set of organs, things went on in my mind—things of which I wasn't aware. That moment, of course, was the most important part of the puzzle, but to label any part as "most important" is not right. It's like an MVP award at the end of the World Series or Super Bowl. Yes, some individual made a great play, had a great game, but it wouldn't have happened without their team. It's never just one person.

Great things happen when people work together. My loving partner Jackie continually exemplified this because she never once gave up. Every single day she stayed with me, a team stayed strong. I would not be here today if it wasn't for her. Jackie took care of me—she still does. The phrase "took care of me" says it all. No other way to put it.

One of the top criteria for getting on the national organ donor list is having an excellent support group. The doctors know from experience if you don't have support, your chances are slim. It's far too large to take on by yourself. Jackie was one of the reasons my transplant team put me on the list. My number one support person—Jackie—the person next to me, helping me, backing me up, was rock solid. Standing right next to her was my daughter Zachera. Between the two of them, the team could see from the minute we met I had powerful support. People ask me how I was able to get through a transplant in such good health. Answer: my unwavering support. My family and friends cared about me and buoyed me at every turn.

Recently, there was an older gentleman at one of our hospital forums who was a "pre" heading into a possible transplant. We got talking and I asked him what his top concern was. He said, "You know, I don't understand much about all this yet, but I'm really worried about this 'support' thing. I live alone, lost my wife three years ago. Only one child who lives in California. Few relatives out East, but...only close friends are a couple of golf buddies. Got some neighbors, but I can't ask them to help; they hardly know me."

As this man described his situation, once again I became acutely aware of just how lucky I was. I had strong people by my side and this gentleman had no one. What would it have been like to try to get a transplant without my dear, dear loved ones?

Someone might ask, "Doesn't this usually go in the back of the book?" Well, it needed to be up front because not only do these people deserve this space, but it will give you an idea of how much love it takes to survive the largest surgery there is. MMHMMM has an incredible lung transplant team staffed by dedicated and brilliant doctors who constantly made difficult decisions so I could live. I wrote a letter to each one of them to somehow show my gratitude. It couldn't begin to touch on how deeply I felt.

A few days after Christmas 2016—the Christmas I wasn't going to make—I sent this:

Dr. Anisee, Dr. Danzer, Dr. Cantor, Paul, Kristen, and Staff,

I'm typing this letter because of my shaky handwriting, and, yes, this is one of Jackie's holiday cards that I didn't send on time. But...well...I wanted to write to you in the quiet hours after all the family gatherings, presents, spreads of food, wine, and cheer moved to memories.

For me, 2017 had a ring to it—a sound I wasn't sure I would hear sixteen months ago. This ring was made up of new thoughts, new hopes, and new friends like you. You all have many patients, you work hard to be good at what you do, and you show up each working day prepared. As it was in my classroom teaching days, it's your job, but please know your job reaches far outward. What you do affects a much larger scope than you probably think about as you walk into MMHMMM on any given day.

I can't explain how vast this "scope" really is, so here's an example:

Christmas Eve afternoon there was a knock on our front porch. I opened the door, and standing there was one of my favorite past students who had just flown to Boyne City from Alaska to be with her family. She's now a professional portrait artist. She handed me a large box with a beautiful oil portrait taken from my daughter's professional photo of me for my HelpHopeLive campaign. Lane carried this three-by-four-foot cumbersome frame in a box through customs at three different entry points, fought with flight attendants to store it, and with a lot of intestinal fortitude, got it safely home to my doorstep. I think I meant a lot to her as a teacher and drama director in her younger years, and she means a lot to me.

What does this story have to do with all of you? The above wouldn't have happened without you. I would not have been there to open the door. Your work is incredibly bigger than you might imagine. I could add many different personal anecdotes...but I think all of you get the picture.

Your work and the work of your colleagues put me on, as Poet Laureate Robert Frost wrote, a road less traveled by, "and that has made all the difference." I am here...thanks to all of you. Yes, it's a big, big picture, but each one of you is an integral piece of an amazing puzzle.

The "scope" thanks all of you...from the bottom of all our hearts.

Robert Emmet

In essence, this letter goes to all the extraordinary people out there who are so deeply immersed in their work they may not fully know the massive "scope" I was referring to. To help my connectivity with other human beings (no, this is not weird), I shake the hands of astonishing and good people whenever I can.

When Jackie and I both graduated with master's degrees in education, there was a line of seated students waiting to receive their doctorate degrees. As we slowly paraded by them, I shook every one of their hands. How many hours did they sacrifice to be there?

Who or what might they save? What cure might they find for a type of cancer? These people and what they do are vastly important to all of us.

If we stop for a second or three, we all can remember or talk about a person who affected our lives in a significant way. At the time, such an act might have seemed small; maybe no one even noticed. But you did. Regardless, the scope is bigger than it initially appeared. Far bigger. It's all of the people who make a crucial difference.

Once, in a private talk with Dr. Anisee, the head of MMHMMM's lung transplant team, I asked her how to handle using real names of doctors, etc., in my book. "I'm in a bit of a quandary. I don't think I'll be allowed to use real names in my book."

Dr. Anisee said, "That's probably best, considering hospital privacy issues and all."

I answered, "Yes, I know, but I wanted you and your staff to get recognition—for people to know the masterful job you all do day in and day out."

"You know, Robert," Dr. Anisee said, "We don't come to work every day to be praised, recognized, or to get our names in print. Although we appreciate the sentiment, we went into this field to heal patients. For the same reason, my staff doesn't want fame either. It's the work we chose, to help people. It's what we do."

I'll never forget Dr. Anisee's explanation. She didn't use the first-person perspective. It wasn't about her. It was "what we do." Her humility was astounding throughout my days at MMHMMM. Considering who she was and the importance of her job as head of one of the top lung-transplant programs in the country, I felt honored just to be in the same room with her, let alone her patient. Dr. Anisee is one of the most incredible human beings I've ever met.

There are remarkable people at MMHMMM. Many of us outside hospital doors have no idea how difficult it is to deal with life and death every single day. I can't even try to capture how stressful and difficult it must be to work with patients and family members who are dealing with the most tumultuous and tragic moments of their lives. For doctors, nurses, and staff, work isn't just sometimes; it's all the time, every day.

The following is a window into the life of one of these talented and amazing doctors. It's an excerpt from neurosurgeon Dr. Paul Kalanithi's book, *When Breath Becomes Air:*

Sometime after midnight, the phone rang. The patient was crashing...I spat out orders. "One-liter bolus of LR, EKG, chest X-ray, stat—I'm on my way." I was the only general-surgery intern on call, my pager was buzzing relentlessly, with calls I could dispense with (patients needing sleep medication) and ones I couldn't (a rupturing aortic aneurysm in the ER). I was drowning, out of my depth, pulled in a thousand directions...I spent the next few hours running between my patient threatening to die in the ER and my patient actively dying in the ICU...I would glimpse my share of death. I sometimes saw it while peeking around corners, other times while feeling embarrassed to be caught in the same room...In moments, the weight of it all became palpable. It was in the air, the stress and misery. Normally you breathed it in, without noticing. But some days, like a humid, muggy day, it had a suffocating weight of its own. Some days, this is how it felt when I was in the hospital: trapped in an endless jungle summer, wet with sweat, the rain of tears of the families of the dying pouring down.

Dr. Paul Kalanithi—one of the leading neurosurgeons in our country—died of lung cancer in 2004. He was only thirty-eight.

Many people never realize what surgeons go through. Unless you know one extremely well or are very close with one, they rarely talk about their work. Many times, surgeons start at five or six a.m. and work throughout the day, with patients backing up because of emergencies. After seventeen hours, they try to head home at eleven p.m., exhausted, only to receive a call back into surgery for another emergency. Some surgeons end up working up to thirty- and forty-hour shifts. Can they say no and let someone die? Their work can be endless. A close friend who is a surgeon told me, "During surgery, you're performing impossibly difficult and detailed procedures while standing. One surgery, I had to stand for fourteen straight hours as my surgeon partner and I struggled to save a man's life. I didn't know if my hands would keep doing what they needed to do."

I asked if the man lived. My friend said, "Yes, he did."

Heroic human beings.

If I wrote about everything, it would take five books. When my daughter Zachera called and told me about the transplant program at MMHMMM, she said, in her exact words, "You'd better get down here ASAP, or I'm going to be really, really angry!" Like her mother, she was going to make me listen. I listened…and my life changed in a magnanimous way.

The word "luck" appears throughout my sentiments, but please understand a major part of the time our real-life luck happens not by chance, but by hard work and massive effort. Luck happens, as it did for me, because of a series of events set forth by diligent, intelligent, and extraordinary people—the same people mentioned above. These doctors saved me, not because they got "lucky," but because of late nights studying, relentless research, long hours of training, intestinal fortitude, physical ability, and caring. They made saving people their life's work.

My letter was about all those people so deeply emerged in and dedicated to their field. Wonder if they know how big their "scope" really is? How far reaching? Why was I lucky? Because of them.

Some people have a problem with gifted programs in schools, special treatment for students who excel, and appropriated money for such programs. This is as opposed to, say, money spent on huge athletic facilities, bussing students who live three hundred feet from their school, or maybe donkey basketball. They say it's not fair to have gifted programs: "Who made them special?" But I always take the time to ask these people one question, "If your twelve-year-old daughter was lying on an operating table dying, would you want a 'gifted' surgeon working to save her?"

6

Theatre Term: "Backstory"

When my words physically showed up on paper so you would know exactly what happened, everything seemed so dark and bizarre. I thought, wait...I could add in some exciting stuff. Yeah, that's the ticket! I could add an ambulance chase scene where spies want lungs for a guy named Bronk in the black market, so they shoot at a sidewinding, siren screeching, super-lung transportation ambulance—which is actually just an ambulance—as it stealthily maneuvers through the shadowy, wet streets of Chicago. Must have been raining. Meanwhile there could be a smoldering sex scene where my stud surgeon is madly in love with this hot, six feet seven nurse in a short skirt but couldn't tell her because his communication skills were lousy, so he wanders around the hospital cafeteria all night eating old, rubbery Jell-O, then decides to hire a biplane to write his newfound girlfriend a note in smoke up in the sky—risky because Chicago's windy—and sure as hell, the letters got jumbled up and spelled out "Howdy Doody" instead of "Will You Marry Me?" So, he gets depressed and eats a whole extra-large tin of Chicago's Barrett's caramel corn. Cheesy mix.

I don't know. Might sell...might not...

Since we're both here, you should probably know a hair or two about me. Sorry about all the "I's." It's autobiographical, so ....

My full name is Robert Emmet and I was born in Detroit, Michigan around 1950. Named after my grandfather, Robert Allen, and my other grandfather, on my mother's side (duh), Emmet Shanihan. Supposedly, my mom picked my name from the famous Irish statesman Robert Emmet. I'm not sure what that was all about, but my mom took being Irish way serious.

Being named Robert, of course, morphed into Bob, which I really dislike to this very day. Bob is boring. Spell Bob backwards, it's the same. Also, Bob didn't fly very well back in the 60s. It was hard to "cop an attitude," to use a '60s phrase, with the name Bob. Friends in my neighborhood had cool names like Sonny,

Jake Man, and TonyOnly. Girls were Sunshine, Cherish, and Sheila. Sheilaaaa not only had a rad name, she had really thick bushy hair, and long dark eyebrows. She looked like she could be the princess of some fierce tribe or something. Sheila had muscles. I never fell in love with her, though. It was weird. At that age, we all fell in love with every single person there was. I mean, yeah. But Sheila, I don't know, Sheila and I were just buddies.

So, hanging out with a name like "Bob"—"Hey, cats, here comes...Bob," was lackluster. Something you fish with. A part on a sewing machine. Something you do with apples floating in water. A woman's hair style, for God's sake!

Therefore—and a big therefore—many of my friends started calling me Em. I liked it. Em was "baaaad." In the '60s, "bad" meant cool. Em was unusual. Em...Eminem way before his time. Even so, most people still call me Bob. I really like Em, though, so I'll use Em here if it's ok with you. Bob/Em...same guy.

Growing up in Detroit city proper—near Livernois and Seven Mile—was more than interesting. Got kicked out of a big parochial school called Hesu in the third grade for skipping catechism class and pushing a cute girl in a mud puddle. Did both, I admit. My friends thought getting kicked out was cool. Pushing the girl in the mud wasn't. I liked her—a lot—which is probably why I did it. Middle-school boys have a strange way of showing their affection. Wrong head is running the show.

When this particular "kicked out" incident occurred, my mom got a call on her turquoise office phone which had a circle dialing thingy and a really long coiled-up cord. (I'm trying to take you to 1959.) The call caused Mom to drive from work and arrive at Hesu, my illustrious Catholic elementary school, in her hot yellow TR3 Triumph sports car. Mom parked right in front of the school and took no time getting into Mother Superior's office. Because she had previous run-ins with Hesu and Mother Superior regarding you-know-who, Mom was primed. My mother was not a happy Hesu parent because of the way her son was treated, and had her Irish dander up before the whole thing even started. Way up.

I'll have to admit, Mom looked pretty sharp as she walked into Mother Superior's dark, musty office. She wore fashionable Peck & Peck clothes, which back then was like Saks, had wavy black hair, was smart, and extremely attractive. Her smile and charm could knock the socks off anyone. I'd watch it happen when she'd talk to clients, which is why she did so well as an interior designer. It was also why Mother Superior didn't like her. A successful business woman in 1959…hmmm…???

But, on this day, Mom was using her charm as an anti-charm on purpose. So, I'm sitting in a hard wooden chair in this creepy old room with this terrible principal thing who had a pure white, starched, cardboard bonnet surrounding her lightbulb-shaped head. She wouldn't stop glaring at me. The kind of glare where people's eyes don't move.

Mom—a.k.a. Ann Emmet, myyyy mom—entered and moved right past me like Beowulf heading into battle. She gave me the look as she went by and then walked straight up to the front of Mother Superior's desk. Mom's ten-point scale was already at eleven. Without hesitating, Mom immediately asked in a stern voice, "Why did you call me out of work? There are all sorts of students in this school. Is my son the onlyyyy student you seem transfixed on?!"

I was impressed. I mean, "transfixed"…wow.

Superior Penguin said, "Since you weren't at home like a mother should be, I had to call you at your supposed work place because your son is constant trouble." Her attitude was more than snippy.

This was mana vs. mana, commando vs. commando, except they both probably had underwear on. At least I hoped they did. Maybe they didn't, and that's why nuns wore those black, cloak-like dresses. Maybe...and this is a stretch...but maybe...it's why my teacher, Sister Mary Herbasite, made me sit under her desk for hours as punishment. Hmmm...

Whilst I was contemplating that disturbing thought, Mom was gaining steam. Mother Superior had no idea with whom she was dealing. Mom raised her eyebrow and said, "My son is constant trouble?" hitting the "tr" hard.

Ol' Mo Superior sat straight up in her big chair and in a gargled high-old voice said, "Your son is a ruffian, a troublemaker. He is retarded and will never learn to read." OMG, she said that...to... my...mother! Yikes, this was getting way out of control, fast!

My mother's Irish temper became Lazarus rising. You could always tell. Mom's face would really flush when she got angry. Her skin was a pale Irish white to begin with, but crimson started filling in her cheeks. "What did you just say?!" Mom shouted, leaning in closer. This was crazy cool.

"You heard me," Mother Superior said, tipping her head side-to-side with each word, which rendered more attitude. Oh boy. The black penguin, head warden of all wardens in Detroit, had just made a fatal mistake. Get smart-mouth with my mother and you were in for it! Mom didn't do "smart-mouth" from anyone. I knew all too well!

Mom's steam was building and directed towards the head of Hesu sitting in her superior chair, "You will not call my son such a thing! Retarded! What a terrible thing to say to a child. You are going to regret that ever came out of your mouth!"

Superior said, "Oh, really. Just what do you think you can do about it?" Oooo, bad question. Wayyyy bad question. I'm sitting in the peanut gallery and I'm thinking, *Don't ask my mother that. I've tried that. Doesn't work.*

A betting person would put big money on my mom at this point. Once her Irish revved up, there was no stopping her. Mother Superior had met her match tenfold and was going to lose her high and mighty attitude "toot sweet" along with her bonnet! Mom's eyes got beady scary as she moved in: "Just what can I doooo about it? In five minutes, I will be on the phone talking with one of my oldest and dearest friends—Father Malcolm Courtney at your archdiocese. I'm sure you know Archbishop Courtney...hmmm? Since he's your...head boss! Right? The head of everything Catholic in Detroit! When I tell him what's going on he'll turn you inside out and backwards. Won't Father Courtney just love to hear one of his top Catholic families is pulling their son out of Hesu because of you!"

Mother Superior looked like she was going to throw up. "You... you can't do that. B...b...besides...you need my signature to... to...transfer...schools, so...there!" As The Penguin continued stammering, it was clear she was way out of her league and fading fast.

In one swift move, Mom turned and forcefully grabbed my arm, pulling me straight up off my chair, deposited me next to the office door, and then turned and headed back towards Mo. I thought, *Ok, wow! Mom's going back to smack Mother Superior and I'll be king of the playground!* I was right about one thing; Mom was far from done. Mother Superior stood up wavering...she was on the ropes.

Mom never backed down in her life—it wasn't in her genes. She took a strong stride towards the withering demon in black and said, with steely eyes and a deep voice, "I am taking my son out of this awful school this very minute, right in front of your fat face. You'll sign a transfer letter, or I'll spread it all over our extremely large Catholic community what you're doing behind closed doors. Discipline!? Let's let everyone know how this school abuses children! I've heard from many parents about duct taping children's mouths shut, hitting them with wooden sticks, and allll about altar boys in the back of the sanctuary! Aaaand, I also know about you and your affair with Father O'Malley!" The knockout punch! Bam!! As it turns out, my mother was wayyyy ahead of her time with a lot of issues! Altar boys!! Father O'Malley and Mother Superior!…whoa…this was like "crazy wow!"

Mother Superior's face went ghastly grey. It was like Dorothy throwing water on the Wicked Witch. Mother Superior was now Mother Guilty, knocked down like Sonny Liston's first round against Muhammad Ali. This time it was Mom hovering over her opponent!

Mom yanked me out into the hallway and slammed the door hard. Mother the Defeated was trying feebly to call Mom back to talk things over. I'll bet she was! Mom never flinched, and down Hesu's front steps I went for the last time. Not sure my feet even touched the ground.

What had just happened was the best of the best! But it didn't last long. As we approached Mom's TR3 convertible, she latched onto my shoulders, swung me towards her, and said, glaring, "Who do you think you are!?" which I always thought was funny because I knew who I was. One time I even answered, "Robert," and all hell broke loose! But this time Mom quickly added, "Don't you think for a minute you're out of the woods, mister!" Needless to say, my euphoria over watching *Thrilla in Manila* faded on the ride home. A new school, unknown students, and who knew what'd happen after today loomed in front of me. As it turned out, I ended up in a predominantly Jewish elementary school called Hampton Elementary—one of the best places this wayward boy could have landed.

"Predominantly" Jewish didn't quite paint the real picture. Everyone was Jewish at Hampton Public School, except this one Protestant girl who kicked a soccer ball a hundred miles an hour right between my legs on the playground on my first day. I was now the new Catholic kid at school with a Princeton haircut.

My school change from Hesu to Hampton turned out to be another lucky break. At the time, Hampton was considered one of the top academic elementary schools in Detroit. Let me tell you, Hesu was below the bottom, and looking up. Hesu had overcrowded classrooms, outdated materials, and very old, hanging-on teacher nuns. Parochial schools were not what people thought they were. There were forty to fifty kids to a classroom, and the only way nuns could survive was to use weird, unusual punishment. I'll bet Sister Magpie still had bits of my skin on her ruler. As I mentioned, she would make me sit under her desk at the front of the class. That was novel at first, but wore off after an hour or two. If I wasn't under her desk, getting my mouth taped shut made for good thoughts during math. Whether it was because of the treatment we endured at Hesu or not, it turned out my Hesu friends ended up in juvenile schools for stealing cars amongst other things. Ironically, my new friends at Hampton Elementary ended up lawyers and doctors... huh.

As I said, Detroit at the time was stimulating. Getting hit by a drunk driver whilst biking down Seven Mile was interesting. I survived by flying ten feet in the air, landing on my ass and not in Seven Mile traffic. Once home, I dumped my sister's mangled bike behind our garage, put a towel on my cut ankle, and got in bed because I thought I'd get a ticket and wanted to keep Mom and Dad from knowing. Didn't work. In fact, it got worse when Dad walked into my bedroom followed by two Detroit police officers. A hit-and-run had been reported and the police were looking for the boy who had been hit. Yep, interesting.

Camping in our city backyard that was like Jack London's wilderness was an opportunity for some late-night hijinks. Lighting a model biplane on fire with firecrackers taped to the fuselage and sending it soaring out my third-story attic window is another story I won't go into. Setting off M-80s in wheelbarrows was fun. And while cooking BBQ ribs with my friends, we left to play street football, and the ribs and my Dad's new grill became so inflamed, all that was left was a solid blob. I could go on and on.

Whilst at my new school, I thrived, and actually—"what-do-you-know!" got good grades in reading! Huh. Guess Ol' Superior was wrong. Funny thing, I never got in trouble either. Well, almost never.

But let me skip ahead to a landmark lucky break that took me down a different road. In eighth grade, playing sandlot football on Hampton's playground—which was actually just a big fenced-in dirt city block—a high-school football coach happened to see me play on a tip from his younger brother. Coach Williams talked to my dad and recruited me to go to Brother Rice High School, a parochial school in Birmingham, Michigan known for top football teams.

Dad told me one evening over a Swift's breaded pork cutlet with applesauce, "Rob, I need to drive you out to a high school your mother and I want you to attend next year. It's called Brother Rice, and, no…it doesn't have nuns." I hadn't heard of it. I was supposed to go to Mumford High School.

My immediate reaction was, "Rice? There's a school called Rice?" Brother Rice High School, an all-guys parochial school, was, and still is, a college-prep high school and a perennial football power. Rice wasn't even close to Mumford. Detroit in the '60s was a tough scene and Mumford had its share of knife fights and gangs. Mom wanted me to go to Rice…soooo, discussion over.

Catholic schools have been accused of recruiting athletes from outside their educational jurisdiction for years. I lived in Detroit; Brother Rice was in Birmingham, more than 20 miles away. Ended up playing three different sports for four years. Hmmm. Later on, while back from Michigan State University, I'd stop by Rice to visit Coach Williams and we'd continue our on-going "recruiting" debate for hours. He helped shape my high school years and was a great coach and friend.

Jackie attended Marian Catholic High School—Brother Rice's sister all-girls Catholic school. Conveniently, it was right next door to Rice. One spring day, Jackie and I met in the median between the two schools. Guys at Rice called it "The Valley of the Dolls." I can just imagine what the Marion girls called it.

Jackie and I dated and then "went together," a saying back in the day, finishing out our high school years. In my senior year, we won the Detroit Catholic League Football Championship and I was recruited to play college football at a number of schools. Our all-state quarterback and I were flown to different colleges to take their tour and sign a letter of intent. Being given big university charge cards for whatever we wanted to buy on that particular weekend was hilarious. But, being madly in love with Jackie, my high-school sweetheart (yes, I can say that because we got married seven years later), I decided playing baseball nearby at MSU was my best option for a scholarship. My reasons: One: because it would put me close to Jackie, who was soon enrolling there, and two: because I was a baseball pitcher and thought MSU would be my big chance to play for the Detroit Tigers. I know, I know, a lofty thought, but, come on, I was seventeen.

Unfortunately, or fortunately, as it turned out, my arm gave out during my first year due to trying to out-throw every pitcher in the universe vying for a spot on the Spartans' roster. Since I couldn't pitch with a bone chip in my arm, I was now on a different path—a path that would affect the rest of my life. While teaching years later, I would always tell my students, "When life puts up roadblocks, learn to maneuver around them." Not that profound, but true. Fighting around roadblocks shaped my future.

One night at MSU, while sitting in my dorm, McDonel Hall, with a messed-up elbow, feeling depressed, and wondering what in the hell I was going to do next, luck blew in. Some call it random, some chaos, some fate. Don't know, call it going with life as it comes along.

My roommate Chip looked up from his desk and said, "Man, you got to stop mopin' around about your bum arm. Go with me to this audition the MSU theatre department is holding tonight. There're a bunch of plays you can try out for."

One was *Death of a Salesman*, by Arthur Miller, which I knew nothing about.

"You're not doing a damn thing right now. Go with me. All the hot women are in the theater department!" Chip said.

"I have a beautiful girlfriend."

"Yah, shmmaaah," Chip quipped, "it'll be fun."

"I've never done any acting."

Chip countered, "Neither have I, but what the hell are we doin' in college if we're not trying shit?"

He had a point. We went and had quite a time. I was picked

to play Biff in *Death of a Salesman*. (Go ahead and laugh, that's the guy's name in the play.) I was probably picked because Biff was supposed to be his dad's sport hero son and nobody trying out looked even remotely like an athlete. Remember, this was 1969 and everyone auditioning looked like John Lennon or Mick Jagger—major long hair, little round glasses whether you needed them or not, overly skinny, neck bandanna, and large bell-bottoms. Very Woodstockish.

Working out all fall with the baseball team, I was in good shape and wore a black t-shirt because I thought theatre people were supposed to wear black. It had shrunk because I didn't know jack about laundry. Sitting in the audience while they called people up on stage to audition, a thirty-something big older guy who didn't look like a student asked me to step out in the hall. Very weird. I was leery. When we got out there, he said, "Look, this is a call for actors for three plays. I'm directing one of them, called *Death of a Salesman*. I need two athletic-looking guys to play Biff and his brother, Happy. I need you to play Biff, the more athletic one."

"Biff and Happy?" I questioned, feeling things were getting mighty murky.

"Yeah. Biff. Have you looked at the students auditioning in there? They've all been smokin' weed since they were two years old. None of 'em fit the bill. Nada. I need you to take the part. Just get up there, read whatever they give you, and I'll yell, 'Got it,' and write you in."

"Look, I'll be honest, I've never been in a play before…and I…"

"Doesn't matter, that's my job as director. You're the guy I gotta have."

Thinking about it, I told him, "I'll take the part if you pick my friend to play…what's his name…the other guy, Funny?"

The director said, "Happy to," and opened the door to the theatre a crack. "Show me your friend."

"He's right there…next to that hot blond chick…plaid shirt."

"Guy with sorta long black hair? Tappin' his foot?"

"Yeah, that's him."

"Is he ok in the head? Not pottin' out or...?"

"He's ok. None of that. Math major."

"Math major...huh...well...alright, deal. But you both gotta audition and make like I never talked to you."

I said, "Deal," and walked back into the small theatre and sat next to Chip. Leaning in, I told him we already had parts in one of the plays. He looked at me like I was zany and said, "What the hell?"

I said, "Dooon' worry abou itttt!" in my best Mafia accent and explained what we had to do. We took the parts, did the show, and both had a great experience. As planned, Chip dated the sexy blond the whole semester.

I'm only writing about this auditioning moment because it has to do with my roadblock theory. After graduating from MSU, I got a job teaching, coaching and, of all things, running a drama department. Do roadblock end-runs enough times, sometimes good things happen.

Years later, whilst teaching one of my AP English classes, my students were discussing Alvin Toffler's quote from *Future Shock*, "The only constant in our lives is change." Throughout my days, I've tried to deal with life as it arrives, good, bad, up, or down. Maybe some people have linear lives. Mine never was. It was all over the place, lots of roadblocks. The main thing was to keep going, keep moving around barriers. I hung on to that theory whenever the winds of change arrived.

After graduating from MSU, I got a job teaching English and coaching at Boyne City Public Schools in northern Michigan because it's beautiful country and they offered me a job for $8,050 a year. Wasn't much, but as they said in northern Michigan, "A view of the bay is worth half the pay."

Boyne City is a beautiful town on the shores of Lake Charlevoix, which opens up to Lake Michigan, so there was that. During my interview, I agreed to teach English full time, coach freshman basketball, cross-country, cover the journalism club and yearbook, and run, as I mentioned, the drama department. I took on this ridiculous schedule because that's how you got a job in those days. Gaining a teacher's job was a major roadblock in the '70s because lots of guys were back from Vietnam, used the GI bill, got a degree, and filled all the teaching positions.

Jackie graduated from MSU a year later, and we got married. We bought a small brick house near the shores of Lake Charlevoix, and Jackie started teaching first grade at Boyne City Elementary School. We ran the drama department at the high school, which turned into a big program thanks to all the wonderful local Boyne City parents, teachers, music teachers, prop builders, painters, and voice and dance instructors. Through my teaching years, I ran the drama department with Jackie, coached baseball, football, cross-country, golf, basketball, whatever our school needed. As a teacher/coach in a small, rural community, you help—end of discussion. Each new year, staff meetings went like this:

Principal reading the list of needs:

"Jenny, you're doing Business Club, right?"

Without looking up, Jenny said, "Yep."

Someone told a joke and the back of the room was laughing and making noise.

Principal says, "Knock it off. Who does baseball? Wollenberg, you played baseball at MSU, right?"

"Yeah, but..."

"Wollenberg, you're baseball coach. Who knows how to play tennis?"

And so it went. Jackie and I spent wonderful years teaching. Along with coaching different sports, as drama directors, our program grew. Jackie, who put in hours and hours of volunteer directing, was finally hired officially as assistant director. By the end of our teaching careers, we had presented thirty-eight musicals, twenty-five plays, and put on a musical revue called *Boyne Meets Broadway* each year. During that span of time, we also did competition productions and took our drama students on thirty-seven different theatre trips to Toronto, Chicago, Detroit, and New York City. We worked with exceptional students, kids who came from great families, broken families, and students who couldn't find any other niche in school for a number of reasons. Incredible young people now out in the world doing great things. We still keep in touch with many of them.

We retired from teaching in 2006-07. Jackie furthered her water-color painting, eventually becoming curator of the Boyne Arts Collective, a nonprofit local artists' gallery. We're both part of this gallery today, promoting art in our community. I started painting soon after my lung transplant because there was a lot of down time, to say the least. After watching Jackie paint for years, I gathered some of her brushes and paint—with her permission!—and gave it a try. Jackie has sold quite a few paintings and I've sold some too, which has been fun and invigorating. Since I've never taken any painting classes, Jackie thinks my new lungs came from an artist. She might be right.

7

Easy Bake, Not So Easy Ride

A few years before coming close to drowning off Glenwood Beach, Jackie and I were spending our beginning days as retired teachers. We didn't have much money as things go, but we had great friends and lived in what downstaters call "the Gold Coast." Somewhere around 2012, I noticed my exercise workouts seemed more difficult than usual. The weights were the same, the time on the elliptical machine was the same, so why was I so tired? Why couldn't I do the same workout? I chalked it up to being in my 60s, allergies, and ignored it.

This went on for about six months, but one fall day Jackie and I were taking our normal afternoon bike ride in Young State Park next to where we live. Biking up a hill heading into the park, Jackie kept getting farther ahead. She's a good athlete and runs lots of miles each week, so I thought she was just pushing the pace more than usual. The trouble was, I could tell I was slowing down. I was trying to keep up, but couldn't. Finally, I had to stop. After a minute or two, Jackie biked back towards me, braked, and said, "What'ssss the dealll!?" which was one of our favorite quotes from Jim Carey's rendition of *The Grinch Who Stole Christmas*.

I tried to cover my lack of energy. "No biggie, just allergies slowing me down. Should probably have Dr. Mike see what's causing them, eh."

Of course I didn't follow up with Dr. Mike, and the days moved on. As they did, my health was turning. Whatever was wrong wouldn't be a big deal, probably something minor. But, as seasons changed, it never cleared up. Jackie would say, "You're coughing an awful lot. What does Dr. Mike think?" My pat answer was always, "Allergies, I don't know. Have to get it checked out." I didn't want it to be serious, so I kept it that way.

Didn't want to see a doctor, but finally Jackie insisted. I grudgingly made an appointment with Dr. Mike, who was actually a past top student of mine and my primary physician in Boyne City. He's also a close, close friend. He knew about my lingering cough. Everyone runs into everyone in a small town. Mike said he'd talked to Jackie quite a few times in the grocery store, etc. She told him about my lingering cough and how my physical ability was starting to decline. When I was sitting on the bench with the waxed paper, he suggested taking a few x-rays of my lungs.

Slightly concerned, I said, "X-rays? My lungs? That sounds ominous."

"Only takes a few minutes. Just a good thing to check at your age," he said. I sensed he was a tad concerned, but went along with the "good thing to check."

Dr. Mike came back in the room and put the x-ray up into that clip holder they all use. Snap. He pointed to a lower area of lungs on the screen and said, "This view…right here…shows some kind of darkness near the bottom of your lungs. Probably nothing, but I think it's worth looking into. I'll get you an appointment with a pulmonary specialist in Petoskey I work with. Let's just have him have a look-see. What do you think?"

Now really concerned, I said, "A pulmonary specialist? What are you thinking it is?"

"Not sure, but it's always good to let someone who examines x-rays of the lung area all day look. It may be nothing at all," Dr. Mike said, in his calm, easygoing way. But, after knowing him for years, my intuition alarm was speaking to me: *He's more concerned than he's letting on.*

After my appointment with Dr. Mike, I carried on with my normal life...like you do. It was fall and the trees in northern Michigan were beginning to show hints of the brilliant colors soon to burst all across Charlevoix County. Dr. Mike did procure an appointment with his pulmonary specialist friend, but it was, like many attempts to get in to see a doctor these days, a month or more "out."

They always say that. Call for an appointment and the secretary will say, "Yes, we can schedule you, but Dr. Fly-fishing's appointments are a good six weeks out, just so you know." Just so I know? Are you saying that so I don't wig out when his next opening has to do with the word "year"?

Deep inside, I knew something wasn't working right. Ignoring it wasn't something I could put aside any longer. This was real. No more avoidance. Jackie was right. She was always right. After going through our near-drowning experience, I had to have Dr. Mike somehow try to get me in to see his specialist. There's a phrase, "scared straight." Although, coming from a completely different scenario, it now applied to me. I was really scared and knew it was time to deal with the fear that was holding me back.

Dr. Mike, as he always did, took care of the logistics and got me in to see a pulmonary specialist right away, claiming, I'm sure, I didn't have time to wait. It seemed like a bit of a favor, but looking back, it was true. I didn't have time.

The results of my CT scan came back, and the pulmonary specialist said there was definitely something there at the bottom of my lungs, and that it could be IPF. Emphasis on "could be." My mother had died from IPF ten years earlier, but since doctors and many national studies claimed there was no link between heredity and IPF, in my mind my mother's illness and what was going on with me was only coincidental. My complete state of mind was that nothing was happening to me and wasn't going to happen, and that was that. Total denial.

Doing research on IPF, I found a lot of evidence of family links as a risk factor. What doctors do say, and I've now had some of the best in the United States, is that even though there is no definitive evidence regarding heredity, they are finding certain groups of

DNAs are specifically prone to one disease or another. This gene grouping shows up a lot with many dangerous diseases and may explain the heredity occurrence, in some degree. They are now thinking the same thing about IPF.

The pulmonary specialist wanted me to immediately undergo a rather invasive test—a surgery where they take out a dime-sized piece of your lung and send it to Mayo Clinic in Minnesota for evaluation. Other than feeling older and thinking age just causes less lung capacity, I wasn't worried and wasn't really feeling sick. Yes, I wasn't twenty-five anymore and wasn't moving around like I used to, but the idea of staying in the hospital and undergoing surgery that dire didn't sound necessary."

I refused. Little did I know then, there were serious issues ahead.

Whether I was in denial or not, whether I was more fatigued than I would admit, I came up with a suggestion that seemed to make sense, to me anyway. I spoke to my pulmonary doctor and suggested, since I felt fine, we wait a year, do another CT scan, and then compare them. If my lung condition stayed the same, then I didn't have anything growing or getting bigger in my lungs, and no big deal. If the CT scan was changed or showed possible IPF growth, we could start with all these serious-sounding procedures. My doctor agreed because he felt there was time to try the idea. If it was IPF, it would—hopefully—take quite a while to get worse. Besides, he said it might be nothing, and there was no way to tell at that moment. Once again, gettin' out of another of life's jams. Buyin' time.

I never liked CT scans. They told a possible story before the possible story had been told, was my stupid and ridiculous thought. I certainly don't think that now. Even so, at that time, I believed it was better to live life to the fullest and suddenly fall off a cliff and become extinct, than to die a long, slow death. People talk all the time about someone they loved: "Paul was such a great guy, but he suffered so when he was ill. He lost one hundred pounds and there was nothing left of him when he passed away." Is that a good thing? Do I want "nothing left of me"? Oh, that was just what I wanted: Someone walking up to my hospital bed saying, "Strange, Ralph was here a minute ago. Wait, what's that under the pillow?! OMG, it's Ralph; there's nothing left of him!" Maybe I wanted all of me around when I died. Sticking with all of me the whole time sounded like a plan. Maybe I wanted people to say, "Gee, he died, but he never lost weight and actually looked pretty damn good." Maybe I wanted someone to say, "We went to the Detroit Tigers game yesterday, walked over to that Coney dog place on Lafayette, ordered Coneys, and Ralph died right in the middle of his third dog." Yep, good plan...but easy to say when you're not seriously sick.

Ten months after that appointment in Petoskey, I was still coughing. Dr. Mike made another pulmonary appointment, but this time the same specialist gave me no way out. He walked in and clipped two different views from my CT scan next to each other on the white plastic screen. Snap. Snap. He said, "If you look at both of these areas," pointing to the middle area of my lungs, "you'll see the honeycombing progression has nearly doubled."

I was in trouble.

"In my opinion, there's no question you have IPF," he said.

There was a long silence. I became uneasy. The walls were closing in on my chances of a way out, a way to get everything back to ok, another way around an extremely large life roadblock. But, to me it still seemed a long way off in the distance. Even though it was right in front of me and it was real, I wouldn't let it enter my mind. Not all the way.

"So...ah...what's next?" I said, truly believing there were just certain steps I had to take and then it would go away.

"Well, they have just come out with a new drug."

I immediately wondered, "A cure?"

"No. There is no cure for IPF. This new drug can slow the IPF progression down, though."

"It slows it down for how long?"

"Studies indicate the drug lowers apex progression, but there are no statistics quantifying the time benefit. It's extremely new. You're under seventy, which is the general cutoff point for lung transplantation, so this medication might be an option to consider."

Truthfully, when this doctor said, "lung surgery," my brain did not go there. Believe me, it sounds as strange as it does writing it, but I did not go there. I wouldn't let it in. I'm telling you the honest truth—I did not accept what he was saying. It wasn't real. This is exactly what happened. Denial, it turns out, is a darker power than we think.

Actually, I had no idea what the pulmonologist was talking about in terms of lung surgery. Maybe there was something in the news I had missed, but all I could think of was patients having tumors taken out, or things of that nature. Maybe it was because Jackie and I only watched the national news occasionally because the media made us depressed. But, honestly, I had never heard of anyone having work like that done. Sitting there in the doctor's office, I wasn't even close to grasping the concept he was talking about. My health was good. I did stuff, worked out, lifted weights. Yes, I could have been in better shape, but we all feel that way.

The same conversation would happen again soon, it turned out, but at that particular time, at that moment, it just didn't register. Looking back, my reaction sort of made sense. To me, it was too early. It wasn't happening. That type of scene is movie kind of stuff. You see it all the time...on film...not in real life...right? Doctor walks in, couple sitting nervously, looks at them with a grim face... the whole nine yards. My mind did not focus on the consequences. *Ok, so I'm legitimately sick, but I can get out of this—eat seaweed, take different pills, exercise more. There will be a way. I'll find a way.*

And I did. It just wasn't what was expected.

Soon, Dr. Mike received the pulmonologist's test results. He called me one morning and asked if I could stop by his office after his last appointment around five p.m. It sounded ominous. We sat down and had a long, serious talk.

After our usual conversation about his family and whether or not he was going to have his collection of tractors ready at the yearly flywheelers show, he got down to business.

"Rob, I received a report from Dr. Winzinski in Petoskey. We've waited a year, hoping to see no further evidence of increased honeycombing in your lungs, but after viewing your recent CT scan, he believes you have full-on IPF and it's getting worse."

What do you say when you hear something like that? I simply said, "Oh." We always picture wild reactions in these situations. A patient jumping up and screaming, "Doctor, no!! It can't be! You're wrong, I know it!!" It wasn't like that. It was just, "Oh."

After a long pause, Dr. Mike said, "If it gets worse, would you consider lung surgery of some kind?"

My first reaction, "I don't know."

He asked, "What are your thoughts regarding going in the surgery direction?

"Well, ah…thoughts…hmmm…well, those special pills made me incredibly sick. Maybe they'll come up with something better. I mean, there's time since this thing seems, from what everyone says, to gain momentum slowly?"

Dr. Mike said, "I'm not sure you have that long. We don't know much about IPF. It's a pretty dark disease, in that there just isn't much we understand. We do know it will progress; it's a matter of how much, how fast."

Cutting right to it, I said, "Where do we start?" It was not what I was thinking, but it was something he wanted to hear. What I was actually thinking was, *we can start all kinds of things, but I'm going to get out of this. I'm going to be fine.*

Looking straight at me, Dr. Mike said, "I want you to be honest with me. We're talking about an incredibly large and difficult surgery. Lungs are complicated; we don't know how it will go. You need to understand that you may not live through it, and, if you do, it will take a long, long time to recover. Are you sure it's something you want to do…you want to go through?"

"If that's what you think I should do, I'll do it. I don't want to die," I said.

We both sat there contemplating that dire thought. Dr. Mike finally broke the silence, "Well, the three top hospitals closest to us are University of Michigan, Cleveland Clinic, and MMHMMM in Chicago. Given your daughter and Ryan live in Chicago, you might want to choose MMHMMM. You would have their support while there and a place to stay. As I said, it's going to be a long, drawn-out process; you will need all the help you can get."

I commented, "Going to Chicago would work. We visit Zachera and Ryan all the time. Picking U of M wouldn't make sense because I'm too much of an MSU Spartan!" I grinned. Mike did his under-grad at U of M and then received his medical degree there as well. Generations of our family went to MSU and we're deeply "green and white." It was a good joke between us and we always kidded each other about it. Sometimes I'd even wear my Spartan jacket and hat to my appointment. He'd walk in, start laughing, and say, "No! Nope! Arrrhhhh!"

Of course, there was no need to react to the news immediately— or so I thought. None of this was going to happen soon, right? There were people to contact, appointments, lots of planning. It was still a maybe, something far off, something escapable. Maybe a new drug to cure it. People went to Canada and Mexico all the time to try new drugs the U.S. hadn't approved yet. My pharmacist friend always says, "Better life with drugs!"

After a moment, Dr. Mike solemnly said, "Rob, there isn't a cure." My mind shouted at me from inside, *That can't be. There is a cure, it's just that mainstream medicine hasn't caught up with it yet*. The FDA was constantly adding incredible new drugs, so a cure was going to show up soon. My pat answer to any problem was, "If we can go to the moon, we can certainly…I can get out of this. There's a way."

The pulmonologist prescribed another new drug called Aspri-yett. After taking it, within a week, the drug made me extremely ill to the point of almost going to Petoskey's emergency room. After that awful set of days, it was obvious the new, experimental drug for IPF was going to kill me before whatever was in my lungs did. I stopped taking it immediately, but my future was becoming murky. If this new drug for my lung problems didn't work, what was next? Narrowing thoughts seeped in like smoke: *This is a deep hole I'm in here.* The strange thing was, I didn't believe it...yet.

Saying I didn't believe it sounds so trite. My close friend and doctor were surely telling the truth. The pulmonary specialist at McCloud Hospital had no reason to tell me something that wasn't backed up by reliable facts. I know it's crazy, but when you're backed in a corner, your mind does some pretty unusual things— especially when it comes to dying.

There was a way out. I wasn't sure Jackie was under the same denial. She was viewing the situation through much clearer glasses, so to speak. We never told our family and friends. We kept Zachera semi-informed with sketchy reports from the doctors because the last thing we wanted was to upset her. She had just gotten married to Ryan, started a new photography company in Chicago, and was swamped with work. All of this was unreal, anyway. I mean, I'd get out of this. I went from thinking it was a stubborn allergy to having doctors tell me it was serious, to the topic of death. But to me the gulf between those views was far too vast. This whole thing took a long time to develop—it would take even longer to get worse. There was no way it could be that bad.

As days flowed by, my coughing became more and more frequent. Jackie and Zachera talked about it between themselves because they knew it was serious and they knew I was in denial... pure, flat-out denial. Finally, after weeks of not wanting to discuss "the problem that didn't exist," Zachera called me on my cell. "Dad, you know you need help. I'm asking you—for me—to do something about your cough. Would you do this for me?"

Taking my usual stance, I said, "I know, I know, it's just going to stop and all this going to the doctor stuff will be a waste of time and money, the usual merry-go-round. Checkups, come in next month, more bills, more checkups. Dr. Mike says it's serious, but I've been like this for a long time. He knows that. So..."

"Daaaad! Listen to me!" Zachera screamed through the phone. It surprised me because she never did that. She was angry and upset. I knew right away this wasn't going to be our normal phone call. Her voice was cracking, and she was almost crying, "You have to come down to MMHMMM right away. They have a top pulmonary department—it's all new—they'll figure this out. You have to call them and get an appointment. I mean now!"

"It will be the same ol' same ol'...They'll say the next appointment they have is in six months. You know that."

"Damn it, Daaaad! I've heard you say that a hundred times! Stop it! This is not something to put off or claim you can't get an appointment for. This is way serious! Get down here. I don't care what you have to do; get down here. If you don't, I'm coming up and getting you. I mean it! We'll find a way to get you in quickly. Mom and I want you to do this. Will you do this for us?" This time it wasn't a question.

Zachera was right. Jackie was right. I had to do this whether I wanted to or not.

"You know, I could call our friend Julie. You know Julie. She was the past student of mine I told you about that did the crazy skating thing."

"Yes, Dad, I know Julie. Of course, I know Julie," Zachera said. She added, "You know that!"

"Ok, ok. I forget shit...Anyway, she works pretty high up in MMHMMM. Maybe she could get me in. She might know someone in the pulmonary department."

"Dad. All I know is you've got to get down here. Ryan and I want you to stay here for as long as it takes. We've got an extra bedroom. Just get down here. Ok?" This time the "ok?" had a lot of emotion behind it. I knew it was time.

"I'll get on it today and let you know what I find out about Julie, promise," I said with a sigh. Ryan and Zachera's place in Chicago didn't really have an extra bedroom, but they converted their work/study room—den—into a bedroom by blowing up two single mattresses for us whenever we visited. They always took care of us and made sure we were comfortable. They never balked at us coming down, either. Yes, we bought them dinner at nice places they knew about, LOL, but, considering they were newlyweds, we were an imposition, no matter how much they said they loved it when we came down. (BTW—"down" is what you call it when you live in northern Michigan and travel anywhere other than Canada...or the North Pole.)

Zachera and Ryan always made our stays fun. We didn't know at the time how important it would be that they lived in Chicago— near downtown where MMHMMM was located—or just how much their converted den with blowup beds was going to mean to us in the days ahead.

8

Great Friends

The phone call to MMHMMM Zachera insisted upon turned out to be fruitful. But just as suspected, Dr. Mike called and said the earliest appointment he could get me at MMHMMM's pulmonary center was close to two months out. All things considered, that wasn't going to work, thus the call to our friend Julie. Julie not only lived in Chicago, but worked in a top position at MMHMMM in the area of heart fibrillation—commonly known as "AFib."

Julie and I hadn't talked in over a year or two. A close friend and one of our favorite students in high school, Julie is a creative, fun-loving woman who brightens up everyone's day. (Alright, I admit, I'm saying a lot about my past students, but we had wonderful students…that's all I'm sayin'.)

Julie and her husband Dan, whom we also taught in high school, had resided in Chicago for years and had done extremely well establishing themselves in a tough, big-shouldered city.

"Julie, this is Bob calling from Boyne," I said on her voice mail. I texted her later to see if she had received my message. Local business friends told me they got fifty or more voicemails a day and never had the time to listen to all of them, so maybe a text would work.

My phone rang around five o'clock and it was Julie. "Heyyyy, how's it going? So good to hear your voice!" she said in her always cheerful way.

93

"Well, it seems I'm always calling you because I need something in Chicago, but this time, it's a really important something," I replied.

"What's up?"

"It seems I've got a health issue with my lungs. Got to see a pulmonary specialist at MMHMMM ASAP, according to Dr. Mike. You know Dr. Mike."

Julie said, "Of course." She knew who I meant; everyone in Boyne knew Dr. Mike.

"More importantly, this call comes directly via Zachera's vehement orders along with Jackie's, so...I kind of have to do it...like right now!"

Julie asked, "Did Dr. Mike call MMHMMM to see if he can get you in?"

"Well, to be honest, that's why I'm calling you. Dr. Mike didn't get far contacting them. You work high up at MMHMMM, and Dr. Mike and I thought maybe you knew someone who could get me an appointment. Things have gotten a bit serious here on my end."

Even though we were friends, Julie stayed true to new medical privacy rules and didn't ask for specifics as to what was specifically wrong with me. "When Dr. Mike called, what did the hospital say?"

"Well, looks like they can see me, but it's going to be at least a month or maybe longer. I'm not sure my lung problem can wait that long. As a matter of fact, Dr. Mike says for sure it can't."

"Oh...that's not good. Let me try to go up to the pulmonary center; I've worked PR with them. Maybe there are some cancellations. I just finished a staff program with them. When are you thinking of coming down?" Julie questioned.

"Yesterday, if they have an opening. Zachera and Jackie are all over me to see someone like 'right now' because I put it off too long. Now, with Dr. Mike's concern, I need to do this. They're worried I'm going to keep putting off my cough and stuff so long it can't be taken care of."

"Let me call you back tomorrow. Maybe I can help," Julie said. Julie always helped—every single time. We talked about Dan, her husband, and what they were both working on, and then, because I knew she was busy, we said a quick goodbye.

Afterward, I thought about what Julie said: "Maybe I can help." Trying to explain and cover how many people helped along my path would take pages and pages. People helped me. Some have no idea how important they were as I traveled through all of it. Sometimes it was the little things that mattered most—a call, an errand I couldn't complete, a friend in Boyne City helping Jackie, best friends driving us down to Chicago in a whiteout snow storm (if you live in a warm climate, you may not know exactly how scary driving in a whiteout can be), a friend watching over our house to make sure the power and heat stayed on. As it turned out, the whole town of Boyne City helped, which I'll explain later.

Julie surprised me with a call the very next morning. "Can you be down here the day after tomorrow? Dr. Danzer, the head of pulmonary, said he could fit you in considering your diagnosis. If you can make it down, have Dr. Mike call Dr. Danzer here ASAP, so your CT scans can be sent directly to his office."

"I'll be there. Thanks, so much Julie." I would say that often to many, many people.

Jackie and I started packing.

This was another moment when time came to a halt—the same stoppage of time as sitting on my living room couch watching President Kennedy's supposed killer. Same kind of time warp. Heading out—staying home. In motion—standing still. Different city, different circumstances, different decade. Time watching quizzically.

Two days later, we arrived safely in Chicago. I will always remember exactly when reality hit me. People talk about being in denial. "As iffff anything like that was going to happen to me!" But in life, facts are facts—no matter how hard you try to slant them (despite what some politicians think…sigh).

Why would anyone deny substantiated evidence? It makes no sense. They do, though. I did…for quite a while. Sometimes our brain works in guarded ways.

I've changed my thinking on denial 100 percent. It does happen, and now I understand why. There are times we blot out things that happen or bury them internally. Sometimes these things are just below the surface, ready to come out. Other times they're deep, deep inside. In the last few years, my transplant situation has changed many of my thoughts, ideas, and much of my overall thinking. A huge perspective shift can do that to you. I'm still changing—every day.

After stopping by Zachera and Ryan's condo in Chicago's Ukrainian Village area to drop off what little luggage we brought, change clothes, and go for a much-needed walk after our six-hour drive, Jackie and I headed downtown. We parked in MMHMMM's patient parking area and entered the hospital's vast lobby. We maneuvered through tube-like connections between many buildings, walked through two overpasses, crossed the Golden Gate Bridge, and finally arrived on the main floor. Next, we had to figure out how to get to Dr. Danzer's pulmonary center office on the nineteenth floor. Elevator directions:

Elevator Section A to floors A1B7 or B9783ZXV are to the right, center, middle, and left, but only on Tuesdays, when we change floor numbers.

Elevator Section B to floors twelve through twenty are above you. Don't try to arrive on floor thirteen because it doesn't exist, but CAN be reached by Elevator Section A.

Offices in the Sechs Building can't be found. Forget about it.

Alright, it wasn't that bad, just seemed like it. We made it to the pulmonary center and a cheery woman met us at the check-in counter. After greeting us with a smile, she asked, "First name, last name, and date of birth?" Some computer clicks later, "You're all set, Mr. Emmet. You can find a seat and one of the nurses will come out and call your name."

Later on, during an employee conference speech at MMHMMM, I spoke about this woman at the pulmonary center as one of my focal points regarding the interaction between patients and staff. Every time I arrived for one of what turned out to be many, many appointments, Marcia was there at the counter. Each time, after our initial visit, she greeted me with, "Hello, Mr. Emmet! How are you doing today?!" She never missed, not once. She had hundreds and hundreds of patients check in, but was always on target with my name, was cheerful, and had my paperwork ready. Maybe this doesn't seem like much; some may even say, "Big deal, it's her job." But she treated me like a human being, she was bright and smiling, and made me feel better about what was going to happen. A small thing? No. Think about it. Why, after all the turmoil and angst I went through, would I remember this one receptionist? Because she cared about me, cared about how I was doing, how I was feeling.

After visiting Marcia, Jackie picked out two seats. Looking around the waiting room was discouraging. Many of the patients were bent over, had on oxygen masks, and some of their coughing sounded familiar. An older gentleman sat to my right. He was dressed to the nines—purple silk shirt, black brimmed hat with a red headband. He had on shiny dress shoes, the kind you wear with a tuxedo. His bow tie was the perfect size. A matching silk handkerchief was stuffed dapperly in his lapel—both were red. He started to address another patient across from him, "Ma'am, are you with God?"

It seemed like a fairly blunt question to ask someone out of the blue. Surprisingly, though, she answered right away, "Yes, I surely am."

The well-dressed man said, "He will carry you across the river. Guide your way."

She nodded, "Em hmm, oh yes, em hmm."

In Detroit, years and years earlier, there was a woman named Ethel who took care of my grandmother. We lived across the street from Grandma on Parkside Ave. I was a teenager and helped my dad take care of Grandma's house, i.e. cutting the lawn, painting railings, taking out the trash, the usual. While helping, I would always take time to wander into Grandma's kitchen to visit Ethel. She always greeted me with a smile and a cold 7UP in one of those little green bottles. We would have wonderful conversations about the Detroit Tigers or how much longer the cinnamon rolls would take in the oven. Important stuff. The same lilt in this man's voice came from Ethel years ago. The same "em hmm, yes, em hmm" inserted next to quickly spoken phrases. Ethel was from Chicago, via Georgia. She would say, "Rob, em hmm, them Tigers gone all to hell...em hmm...caaan't hit worth a dog! None of 'em." My dad told me, "She's taken care of Grandma and Grandpa for a long, long time. Been extremely lucky to have her help."

Sitting in the waiting room listening to the woman across from us speak took me back to Ethel, a wonderful, strong woman. A woman who cared for others.

A nurse came through the swinging door. "Robert, Mr. Robert Emmmmetttttt?" holding on to the last syllable. Thoughts of Ethel, homemade bread, and Grandma's kitchen faded away.

When we got up, the nurse said, "Right this way, please," and took us into what reminded me of an inner sanctum—quiet, no one talking. There was someone coughing, though, and a low hum coming from some type of machine. We wound past room after room. Some had patients, some didn't. Farther down, patients moved along with walkers, slowly. As we came closer, they nodded silent hellos, and we moved by them. Many were old and looked very, very tired.

"This is your room," the nurse said. "Dr. Danzer will be in shortly," she added, flipping out an orange metal sign that was hinged and moved back and forth. It was one of four signs alerting staff we were in the room and probably gave the reason why in a type of code. This is going to sound strange—keep in mind how out of sync our whole day was—I imagined the flip-out, metal signs meant, "Green: Probably ok...Blue: Might be ok...Orange: Pretty messed up...Red: Might die before appointment starts." Sorry, just my thoughts. Hadn't been to a doctor's office like this one in quite a while, other than to fix my sixteen-year-old old broken arm or get a crazy colonoscopy. My frame of mind was in right field.

Soon there was a knock on the door and Dr. Danzer stepped in. (They always knock so they don't walk in on you picking your nose or stepping out of your underwear.) Dr. Danzer was medium height, slender, and had the usual white coat with his name monogramed on the front. He had an Indian accent and was very soft spoken. After introducing himself, he explained in very precise sounding English what the pulmonary department was and the different health issues they treated. He asked friendly questions about the two of us and told us a few things about himself. He quickly turned our conversation towards my health and the background behind my coughing. He had read Dr. Mike's file and wanted to know what we thought about it.

Jackie and I both relayed what our lives had been like lately and how and why we had ended up at MMHMMM. He kept nodding his head, saying, "I see," in a quiet voice.

Finally, he said, "This is good you tell this. It gives much better picture of what is going on regarding your breathing, Robertttt. How do you feel today, right now?"

"Well, I guess the same as I have for quite a few weeks now—tired, not able to walk upstairs without being winded, that sort of thing. Other than that, I don't feel particularly sick. Jackie and my daughter, Zachera, hear me coughing a lot, especially at night, so they're concerned. Of course, I am too, but I keep hoping it's allergies. Figured it couldn't be really bad or I wouldn't be able to do anything at all, right? I guess that's why I'm here, to find out."

Dr. Danzer thought for moment, "I viewed both CT scans your primary doctor sent me early this morning at some length. If you wouldn't mind waiting, after talking to you both just now, I'll take one more careful look at them and be back to talk. This acceptable to you both?" He was so polite.

"No problem at all," I said, looking at Jackie. She smiled her beautiful smile. She was next to me. She had ahold of my arm. She would be next to me...the whole way.

Dr. Danzer spoke in short, crisp, but comforting words, "Then, back shortly and we talk." And he got up and left the room.

Whilst waiting, Jackie and I talked about the rest of the day, what we were going to do. There were six hours left on the parking voucher the hospital gave us, so maybe Jackie could stroll

Michigan Avenue. She always enjoyed shopping there because it's one of the best areas to shop in the Midwest. No bargains, but top companies. We spent many a weekend around Christmastime viewing Macy's window displays, eating Frango chocolates, and having lunch at the Grand Lux above Ann Taylor.

We discussed how long my appointment would take and things Dr. Danzer might need, whether there were things we didn't know, and, if necessary, where we would stay if all of this was going to take more than a day or two. Ryan and Zachera had only been married six months. The last thing they needed were parents doing a long sleepover. How long would we be in Chicago?

Another knock and one of the nurses came in and checked through a lot of paper work: full name, address, email, favorite movie, preferences for pizza toppings. Then Dr. Danzer knocked, entered, and sat down. The nurse quickly slipped out.

"Jackie, Robertttt. I compared both of your previous CT scans and it is clear to me you have advanced IPF. Would you possibly be free this afternoon to meet our lung transplant team? The team meets on Thursdays—which is today—so this would be a good thing."

All of a sudden, the mention of a lung transplant was real. In northern Michigan, it was just a theory, a guess, something distant, something unreal. Because one of the top lung specialists in the country was now talking about a lung transplant—a lung transplant involving me—time halted. It just stopped. Now was staying right where it was. There was such a sense that nothing was moving forward, like a bullet stopped in mid-air.

"What you're saying is...we should meet your lung-transplant team because you think I might need one?" I asked incredulously. Dr. Danzer didn't say anything, just looked at me like he wasn't sure what I meant. I said, "You mean...if I don't get a lung transplant there's no other plan? Lung transplants? You can do that?"

Dr. Danzer said quietly, "Yes, we can. "

I looked at Jackie and turned back to Dr. Danzer, "What will happen? I mean, do we have some time here? You can do something like that…like…now?" I asked. Thinking back, I always used the word "we." I immediately included Jackie in my situation. It was as if I hadn't ever given her a chance to decide or even a choice.

"From comparative CT scans, the IPF growth in both lungs has been rapid. IPF is disease that needs study—we don't understand at this point. Disease seems to plateau and then plummet." He paused. "No reason. The latest growth indicates your IPF is at an advanced stage. From what I view, you might have year, maybe less. Please understand, there is very little data of your situation. Picking how much time to an unmanageable stage is, truthfully, educated guess. Please know this. Please. I wish there were more definitive answers."

"You're saying I might die?"

There it was…in front of me. It finally hit home. It was finally real. So many months had gone by where I was sure I could get out of this. Maybe it was something else, maybe they just didn't know. Doctors make mistakes. Hospitals mix things up. But there it was. A top specialist was sitting with me explaining that I might die. My avoidance, my fantasy, my rosy-colored glasses fell apart, and pieces shattered on the floor.

In an almost dazed way, I asked, "A lung-transplant team?" That's the way Hollywood always portrayed someone getting difficult news from a doctor, right? The dazed look, the "could it be?" It was just so strange being in that scene for real—having it happening to me. Where were the cameras? Where was the script? When did we get our break before shooting the next scene?

All my life, death was always clouded, vague. Of course, it happens. I knew that. Everyone knows that. But it worked so well to place it on a shelf in the basement the same way you stored unused household items. We might use them sometime in the future, so we didn't want to throw them away. How often do we think about our own death? When we attend funerals, we probably think about it. Maybe not. It's uncomfortable. Thinking about such abstract notions messes with your mind. Better to close the cabinet door, go upstairs, and tend to it later.

I wasn't thinking or saying anything, so Jackie offered, "We can definitely meet the lung team this afternoon, doctor. Where would you like us to go?"

My mind whirled back to Jackie's voice, the office.

Dr. Danzer stood up. "The nurse will come right back and explain details. Sorry couldn't give better news, but I think this…this may be good thing, a chance." We shook hands, he nodded to Jackie, and said, "Very nice to meet, and see you this afternoon." Then he left. Our lives had changed just like that.

Jackie's eyes had welled up. I said, "It will be ok. We'll just go to this meeting and listen to what they have to say. We don't know." But I knew. This was as real as real gets. The only way to beat my IPF was now on a pathway to something called a transplant. Not wanting to make Jackie more upset, I didn't tell her what was sinking deep inside me. For lack of a better way to put it, the gig was up. All my end runs were over. I might die. I might die within the year. If we chose a lung transplant, I might die from the difficult and intense surgery. I wasn't going to be able to talk my way out of this one; no alternative thinking, being creative, no "there's a way." This was it. This was far too serious for that kind of thinking. If I didn't do this, I would die. It was on the table. When a roadblock presented itself, an alternative could be found—but not this time.

A nurse came in with instructions regarding the lung transplant team's meeting and where and when we should arrive. She said, "You can go now. The halls are a bit confusing, so I'll show you how to get out."

But I couldn't get out. Not out of this. Not this time. My mind kept it up. There was always a way, some way…but not now. I finally admitted the truth. I let it inside…it was big and dark and started taking up room within me…I was going to travel on a journey, a serious, serious journey…a journey that might end before I wanted it to.

9

Prelims

It was that quick. Zachera took an Uber downtown to meet us at the hospital. She had been worrying all day about my appointment, and I knew, since we were headed into something far more dire than we initially thought, she would want to be with us.

We walked into MMHMMM's lung transplant office and met a woman at the desk, Stacey, who would be one of the individuals I'd work with throughout my ordeal. She immediately took us down to a conference room with a long table surrounded by business chairs on rollers. The three of us had no idea what was going to happen next. All Stacey said was that different members of the MMHMMM transplant team would be coming down to meet us.

After Stacey left the room, I looked around and said, "Well, this is going to be interesting."

Zachera said, "I'm not sure we'll know much today. I think this is just preliminary stuff. Hell, I don't know. Who knows! This is all so crazy surprising."

"I know," I said, and added, "We certainly didn't know this was going to happen when we called Julie." Zachera looked at me.

Jackie wasn't saying anything. She turned back and forth in her swivel chair and finally said, "Dr. Danzer said he wanted you to meet the team, so it's probably, as Zachera says, preliminary whatever."

We sat for a while in silence. Talking about anything seemed superfluous.

"This is pretty crazy," I mumbled. The term "crazy" kept popping into my head because it was the only way to think about it. It was crazy. We had driven down to Chicago the day before, had dinner with Zachera and Ryan, and all of a sudden, we were meeting with a lung transplant team. Who ever heard of that?

Stacey walked back in with a young woman wearing a white lab coat similar to all the medical employees moving around the massive hospital. She had blond hair, sharply cut bangs, studious black glasses, and held what looked like a clipboard. A few pens were fastened on the side. She also had pamphlets and other magazine-looking booklets I assumed were going to be given to the three of us explaining how easy and simple all of this would be... or, realistically, not.

Stacey said, "This is Kristen, and she's a head nurse with the transplant team. Kristen will start explaining things, and other members of the team will be in shortly."

"Hi. You're the Robert we've heard so much about," Kristen said.

Obviously, she had some information about me already. I wasn't sure how, but that didn't matter. I was impressed. Jackie said, "I'm Jackie, Robert's partner, and this is our daughter, Zachera."

"Pleased to meet all of you," Kristen replied, "Did you drive all the way from Michigan today?"

I answered, "No, actually, we drove down yesterday and stayed at Zachera's and her husband Ryan's house in Ukrainian Village. It's not too far from downtown."

Kristen said, "Funny, that's near where I live. Love the brownstones in that section of the city, because each one is so different." Then, shuffling some of the materials in front of her, she said, "Well, we've got lots of things to go over, so I should probably get started."

Kristen outlined how MMHMMM's lung transplant team was set up, and the team's present status in terms of patients. We covered a lot of ground, but what stood out immediately was the team was fairly new, having pulled top doctors and surgeons from all over the United States. Other hospitals were doing lung transplants, but MMHMMM was building a dream team, so to speak, of excellent surgeons for lung transplantation. They had only performed nineteen lung transplants, whereas other hospitals known for lung transplants performed fifty to one hundred per year. MMHMM was attempting to be one of the top programs in the country.

Different team members came in the room and sat with us at the large table. They introduced themselves and each explained their specific role on the team. While we were talking, I noticed a small, slight, dark-haired woman standing quietly in the back of the room. Like the rest, she had on a white lab coat with pens in her upper pocket. She stayed there for quite a few minutes and seemed to be listening intently. When she saw me looking towards her curiously, she walked forward and quietly interrupted our conversation, which seemed totally fine with Kristen. In a slight voice she said, "Hi. I'm Dr. Anisee. Sorry to interrupt, but I wanted to meet you, Robert." Between Kristen's "we've heard so much about you" comment and Dr. Anisee's, "I wanted to meet you, Robert," I was feeling kind of honored, in a way. A guy from a small town in northern Michigan now in a city of five million people, it seemed strange to be someone they wanted to meet. It made me feel better, which I'm sure was their plan.

Kristen quickly announced, "Dr. Anisee is the head of our lung-transplant team. She runs our entire program."

Dr. Anisee quickly added, "If you don't mind, I'll just sit here in the back. I do have an appointment shortly, but I thought it would be good to meet all of you and listen in."

Little did we know our entire meeting was actually more like an interview. It was obvious this was a lot bigger deal than expected. Our introduction to the transplant world now seemed more like a science fiction novel than the office visit envisioned. For this staff, our meeting/interview was obviously high stakes. Way high stakes. Everything was beginning to, as they say, "amp up." An incredible amount of work was going to go into each decision they made. They were taking in every word we said, evaluating our attitudes, our relationship to each other, our circle of friends, how we each felt about a transplant, what questions we had. In short, whether I would be a positive candidate for their transplant program.

One comment made whilst we talked stuck out above others. Kristen said, "You need to understand we only accept around five percent of the patients we meet. There's a long, tedious process of tests you have to go through before we even know if you qualify for a transplant."

The roller coaster. I was feeling so good about everyone we were meeting. They seemed so interested, surely they would say, "You can check in tomorrow and we'll get started." I couldn't have been further from the truth. My heart started to sink. This wasn't at all what I'd thought. This wasn't going to be something I just breezed my way into and back out.

Other team members arrived, including Dr. Danzer, the doctor we met in our morning appointment. We had quite a discussion centering around my background and my latest health issues, but interestingly it was mainly about Jackie, Zachera, Ryan, and other family and friends who made up my support group. The team seemed very interested in knowing who would be able to assist me if we did indeed end up being accepted into their lung-transplant program. I thought we would be giving out typical information like phone numbers, addresses, and doctors' names, but the team paid more attention to more personal aspects. They asked about Jackie's background in teaching, Zachera's life in Chicago, where we went to school, and how we ended up at MMHMMM. It seemed to be more of a group talk than an interview, although I knew they were certainly listening and watching for much more.

We touched on some serious subjects. They asked us how we felt about transplants and what our perceptions were. I was embarrassed to tell them I didn't know lung transplants even existed. I mean, I knew there were different types of transplants, heart, kidney, etc., but I had never zeroed in on lungs. It was still a shock that we were sitting talking to them at all, let alone discussing something as huge as a lung transplant.

The team explained how patients are chosen for their program, how donor lungs got distributed nationally when they become available, and how things would proceed if I was chosen. How, once accepted, I would be given a score by the national organ donor program, which would determine when and if I might be given new lungs. What made up your score were things like age, severity of condition, overall health, attitude, and support.

There would be a series of tests to go through to qualify. I immediately asked, "What if I don't pass a test? Does that mean I'm out; I can't get a lung transplant?" There was no way of knowing then the vast array of tests the team was actually talking about.

Kristen replied, "If any tests come back problematic, our team will evaluate the problem and whether or not it will keep you from moving forward. Some issues can be corrected, but, of course, doing so would put you further behind in terms of your position on the donor list."

I said, "In other words, if I don't do well on one of the tests, like something shows up that can't be fixed, I'm out. Yes?"

Kristen came back with, "Not exactly. It depends on a lot of different factors. That sounds odd, I'm sure, but it's the way it is. We can't afford to use healthy donor lungs on a patient who might soon develop or already have other compromising circumstances."

I nodded and said, "I see." I'm not sure I did see, but it seemed to all make sense.

Dr. Anisee said from the back, "I have to go. I would love to stay, but I have patients waiting. It was so good to meet all three of you. Kristen will finish discussing what comes next. Talk to you soon."

Jackie and Zachera both said, "thank you" at the same time, and out the door Dr. Anisee went. Kristen got up as though we were finished, but then said, "Our clinical psychologist, Mr. Paul Schroeder, should be here shortly. He will talk to you about certain issues and then you'll be able to go. Thanks for coming today, and, as Dr. Anisee said, we'll be contacting you soon." Kristen gathered up her folders and left the room.

We sat still for a minute. Zachera finally turned and said what all three of us were probably thinking, "Wow, didn't expect this. I had no idea it would be like this."

Jackie added, "I know. I didn't either."

I sat quiet for a minute as we waited to meet the next team member. Then I said, "It all makes sense...to go through all this. I mean, all the tests. What they're talking about. I guess a lung transplant isn't your average operation."

A tall, lanky young man came through the door, walked right up to us, and said, smiling, "Hi, I'm Paul, and I'm the team's clinical psychologist. I'm the one the team will ask if you're a good guy or not! Just kidding."

Paul certainly broke any ice that existed right away. This was always something he did whenever we worked with him—he made you feel instantly comfortable. He proceeded to ask about each one of us, starting with Zachera, which surprised me.

"Ah...Zachera, I see you're a photographer in Chicago?" Paul commented.

Zachera described her company and what exactly her work entailed. "I do mostly wedding photography, but also family shoots, events, and sometimes company head shots, etc."

Paul asked, "Do you work every day or at different times during the week or month?" Obviously, he wanted to know how available Zachera would be for help if I went through with the surgery.

"It depends on the job," Zachera said. "Some days I spend time at home editing my last shoot, and sometimes I have to travel long distances, even to different states. Since it's my own company, I control my schedule, which is nice."

"Sounds like a cool job," Paul said.

We talked casually and Paul mentioned to Jackie that the information we had filled out prior to arriving said she had been a teacher for thirty-eight years. Jackie said, "Yes," and that was it.

I knew this whole hospital thing—my thing—was going to be difficult for her all the way around. She disliked everything about hospitals—doctors, checkups, needles, the works. Jackie had only been involved in anything medical when she had Zachera, and that had not gone well. Mr. Paul was going to find it challenging to get Jackie to say much.

"What are your thoughts about Robert going through a lung transplant?"

Jackie said, "I don't know much about it, so I really don't have any thoughts yet." Right to the point.

Paul said, "You must have some thoughts about all of this?"

"I do, but I'm going to wait until I know more," Jackie replied. She was saying exactly what she was thinking. That was Jackie. No one pushed her into a corner. In a hospital or around doctors, she immediately felt threatened. Hospitals can do that to you.

Paul finally turned his attention to me. His questions, again, were surprising. I thought he'd ask about my lungs and how everything had gotten to this point, but he was more interested in where we lived, what we did in a small town, and our friends. We didn't know it at the time, but having a strong support group around us was one of the hospital's top criteria. It was what they were looking for. As things moved on, I soon found out why.

Paul finished explaining specific parts of the program and then said, "I'll be contacting you in the next few days regarding the team's decision to accept you or not. Many factors enter into the equation. It will take time to compile everything from Dr. Danzer's report, your CT scans, our notes, and, of course, Dr. Anisee's overall evaluation. Please understand the team will do all it can to help you."

He stood up and asked us if we'd like a soda, coffee, or some water. Jackie chose water, which she always did. She stayed in good health and drank water constantly. As for me, drinking a lot of water rather than a liter of Pepsi was going to be a new, learned experience. I'm happy to report my diet soda days are over.

Three days later, on a special Thursday evening, Dr. Anisee called. "Robert?"

"Yes."

"This is Dr. Anisee from MMHMMM."

"Hi. How are you doing?" which was a dumb thing to say, but my usual pat answer.

"Our lung transplant team met this afternoon," she paused. "After going through your files, we think you would be a strong candidate for a transplant."

Her words took my breath away. I couldn't believe what I was hearing.

"You mean I can start? I really can?" My comment didn't exactly match what was going on in my head. It sounded like a good thing to say, but was I really going to do this? "A strong candidate"? My mind whirled. How do I know if I'm strong enough? Could it wait? Should it wait? Would Jackie, Zachera, and Ryan be ok with all this? It was so bizarre because...I was over-the-top happy to hear Dr. Anisee's words, but her words meant it might really happen. It was right now.

"Yes," Dr. Anisee said. "Robert, you have an exceptional attitude, an extremely solid support group surrounding you, and, if you can pass the testing we have to perform, you are the type of patient who can be successful."

"Dr. Anisee, I can't thank you enough. I can't wait to tell Jackie and Zachera."

"Mr. Paul Schroeder will contact you regarding appointments. He'll be the one to get you started. We'll meet soon. Take care."

If we even said goodbye, it got by me. This was a turning point. My heart finally settled back where it needed to be—in a good place—and I wiped the tears from my eyes. This was so hard to comprehend. My emotions were all over the place. Everything went so fast. Driving down from northern Michigan, I was mired in dark thoughts of dying. I didn't say anything to Jackie, but death was tailgating our car and I knew it...Now I was being told I might have a chance. But it might take miracle surgery. It might not go well. Thoughts raced around in my head.

I took a deep breath and slowly let it out. This was all so, so much. No matter, I had to tell Jackie right away. I was being given a chance...a chance to live.

10

Checkbook Reality

From November to December 2015, MMHMMM's lung transplant team put me through test after test to see if I was eligible for the national donor list. Zachera spent a lot of time Googling what was going to happen if I made it through all the tests and was actually put on the national organ donor list. There were so many elements to consider: timing, long-term lodging, transportation from northern Michigan to Chicago, local transportation in downtown Chicago from hotel to hospital each day and back, meals, groceries, pharmacies, how much time Ryan and Zachera would need to take off work to help when it got close, and, one of the major issues—finances. I was looking at, on average, three to six months or longer to wait for donor lungs if I was lucky enough to get them.

Once lungs were found, average time for full recovery from double-lung surgery was all over the place. If recovery went well, it could be three or four months. Possibly longer if there were any complications. At first, I would have to stay very close to the hospital working with my lung team. The cost of lodging alone for that many months was staggering.

Zachera and Ryan knew help was needed in many ways, and it was clear, if I went through with this and was lucky enough to be chosen from the national donor list, we'd have to discuss finances. The overall cost and magnitude of a double-lung transplant—one of the largest surgeries in terms of size in all of medicine—would be astronomical. If I was lucky enough to be given donor lungs and went through with the transplant, how were we going to afford it?

This, of course, seemed like a moot point. Of course, I would go ahead with a transplant if given the chance. It came down to: lung transplant—possibly live.

No transplant—die within a year from IPF. Why would there be a question? People use the phrase, "a no-brainer." Not quite. Let's just say there was a lot more for my brain to consider than first met the eye.

Ethics will come up in later chapters, but, for me, when all this consternation was happening, there was a type of ethics umbrella hanging over me. It read, "I've lived my life...maybe it's time to move on." My thoughts continually ran towards, *Am I worth such a huge undertaking?* I wasn't being self-deprecating at all. It sounds like it, but I wasn't. It was a major internal conflict between wanting the chance to live on, even while knowing it would take herculean efforts by those surrounding me...or just living out my life the last few months. Tough concept to work through, and on my mind constantly.

My parents taught me to never want anything. They taught me to appreciate everything I had. "You know, there are a lot of kids out there who would love to have what you have. When you stop whining, think about that for a while!" I had wonderful parents. Living life with the concept of not wanting made me appreciate everything that came my way. I never took things for granted. It kept me happy.

Because of these viewpoints, thoughts turned within me. *I've had this extraordinary life. I couldn't have been luckier if I tried. And, now, I'm going to ask my family, friends, and a huge number of professional doctors, nurses, and staff at a major U.S. hospital to give all their attention to ME.*

I spent days secretly mulling over the situation. It didn't escape me. The trouble was, I knew both sides made sense. One just seemed selfish.

There were so many factors to consider, my head was a Tilt-a-Whirl.

I couldn't prioritize one over another. If I went ahead with a double-lung transplant, it immediately put a gigantic burden on Jackie. She would have to go through each and every day with me in dire straits—tubes, walkers, etc. I don't need to explain. Jackie would be in it whether she wanted to be or not. No, she didn't have a choice because she is the most true-blue human ever born. She stood by me my whole life and I knew she would be by my side no matter what, and her "no matter what" was very, very strong.

Zachera's daily life would be greatly affected. She was newly married and both she and Ryan were trying to carve out their own careers and lives. The last thing she needed was an apple cart as upset as my situation would prove to be. Ryan had a new job, and, as it is whenever anyone takes on a new position, there was a voluminous learning curve, many long hours of work, and a great deal of stress.

Don't get me wrong; Jackie, Zachera, and Ryan were never afraid of hard work. Even though I had a parental viewpoint, there was no question all three of them would work hard. Their careers would keep going. That wasn't the issue. What it boiled down to was—should I put my burden on them? On everyone? What if a transplant didn't work and I got worse? Such a scenario would complicate things tenfold. What if I end up bedridden, incapable of doing normal tasks? That reality was sobering at best. It was a catch-22.

We're taught and believe in never giving up, fighting until the end. Going through with a lung transplant would follow from those beliefs.

But not wanting to ever hurt or burden others is admirable. *Maybe I should let my body take its course.*

As a close friend of mine likes to put it: "What to do?" We use this on Friday nights when our friends discuss where to go to dinner together. This choice, however, was of a much different magnitude.

Staring at the financial picture alone was daunting. Being retired teachers from the Michigan public school system, Jackie and I had saved as much as teachers could. Jackie spent much of her paycheck on her students throughout her career, buying supplies the school didn't provide, purchasing a small library of books on her own for students right in her classroom, and paying for small field trips in the local area the school wouldn't monetarily support. We spent money taking drama students to bigger cities, to universities, and helping student athletes throughout my coaching days in any way I could. In short, we didn't make much money teaching. We had a long-term savings, but it didn't involve a lot of digits, so to speak. We loved our careers, our students, and never, ever regretted our decision to go into teaching back in the day. It was just that now, faced with a mammoth health problem, money— whether I wanted it to be or not—was a major factor.

Teachers' insurance was adequate—not great—but it had worked out throughout our teaching years and seemed to be ok when we retired, but neither of us had ever been seriously sick. Now we were entering uncommon ground, and Jackie and I had no idea where a double-lung transplant operation was going to take us in terms of cost, let alone the peripheral bills and charges over and above the actual surgery itself.

Zachera contacted quite a few programs—some state, some federal, some private—for help with the type of situation I was soon to be in. She ran across a wonderful project called HelpHopeLive that sets up fundraising programs for patients with life-threatening diseases. Zachera immediately set one up for me and, thanks to all of my family, close friends, past students, and the unique small town of Boyne City, Michigan, Jackie and I were able to weather the storm, as the saying goes.

Once again, because of HelpHopeLive and my home town, I was incredibly lucky. But there was still the unknown. There were far more roadblocks than I even wanted to envision. I knew that. Reality—what was really going to happen— was a murky road.

A few friends did make the comment when I first found out I had IPF, "You'll be ok, you have insurance." It was a lot more complicated than that. What's covered, what's not? There were non-medical costs: hotels, travel from northern Michigan to Chicago, meals, rehabilitation. Some procedures are blatantly denied, some pharmaceutical costs are questionable, some are not covered at all.

The looming question was, where were we headed with this financially, and would Jackie and I lose our whole life savings going through with it?

We had covered this "late-in-life health and what might happen" discussion throughout the years. I think we all do—it's a dark discussion—but the reality of when you're going to die is part of living. We had worked too hard making our life to lose everything because of health and state laws governing estates, our home, and retirement savings. We had spent years in college gaining degrees which cost not only in tuition, but lodging and other expenses involved when going to school and working part-time. We never made any significant income in four years working part-time. Part-time pay never stayed even with the rise of college costs. Our degrees only took four years. Today, college students take an average of five years to complete a bachelor's degree because requirements have gone up and it's much harder to get into certain programs.

A four-year college degree, on average, at $25,000 per year, equals approximately $100,000. Wages lost by attending class and not working represent $25,000 per year, or $100,000 over four years. Because of this, a college student has a combined cost of about $200,000 over four years. It's actually much higher if you factor in costs I haven't mentioned.

Decisions and paths you take throughout your life affect it every step of the way. I only mention this financial breakdown because it's important. Many times people don't realize it took a lifetime to build a savings, put together careers, build or buy a house. We bought each two by four for our house with money left over from our monthly paycheck. We carried wood, pounded nails, pushed up walls, and laid down roofing. Our friends helped. We brought up a wonderful child, put her through high school and eventually college. It's all a big deal, a really big deal. And, it's not something you throw away after forty or fifty years of work. Some say, "It's only money," but it's way more than that when you sit back and look at it as a whole, as a lifetime.

Deciding to move forward and live or let life take its course was formidable. Such a decision involves quality of life. It's why you spend your whole life working: to take care of your family, to make sure they have a decent life, to make sure in your older years you're secure, to make sure your family is secure. It's real. One decision makes it fairly simple—the other makes it much more complicated. Ultimately, it was up to me.

I wanted Jackie to live in our house, not have to sell it. We'd lived in our house for forty-five years. Maybe she'd want to move and be closer to Zachera in Chicago. She needed to have the ability and money to make that move, to travel where she would like, to have a life of her own. We both worked too hard to have our family racked with bills, taxes, and struggling to make it to the end of the year.

My health wasn't going to eat up everything we had. After thinking about this quagmire, it became evident my life had been everything I had wanted it to be. I couldn't have asked for more. There had to come a time when it ended because life doesn't go on forever. If my body failed me, I'd fight back...but, I didn't have to. It was my life and I'd do what was needed. What wasn't happening was someone else telling me what to do. I refused to let my life drag down my family.

I didn't talk to anyone about it. We all think about our mortality privately from time to time. Throughout my teaching years, I knew my dad had heart problems, etc., and that hereditarily I wasn't going to live forever, either. I helped my dad when he was sick and finally died. My mom developed IPF three years later and died from it. Jackie was with me through all of it. It was difficult, and it was proverbially writing on the wall for me as well.

So, the health thing was real and a fact of life. Now, because it was coming much closer than mere speculation with the onset of my IPF, I kept mulling the situation over and over in my head. One night I finally decided to have a long talk with Jackie. It was after dinner and we had settled in the living room to read or watch TV.

Jackie was sipping her tea, snugged up in blanket on our big lounge chair, legs tucked underneath, her long hair curled, as always, down her back. She was beautiful sitting there so quietly. "Jackie?"

She looked up. "What?"

"Can we talk about something?"

She never liked it when I asked her if we could talk. She always knew it was going to be something serious and probably something she wasn't going to like. It was the same for me when she called from the kitchen in a loud voice, "Robert!" I knew I had either left the milk out all night or some dastardly deed. If she used "Robert" instead of "Hey" or "Hon," I was a goner.

"Yep. What do you want to talk about?" she said, because she always listened.

"Looks like, if I'm lucky, I could be put on the lung donor list. If that happens, we're headed into some crazy times. But there's something I want you to know."

"What?" She never liked "what ifs."

"I'm sixty-six and have had an incredible life. If this whole lung-team thing doesn't work out, I want you to know it's ok. I mean..."

She looked at me with a blank expression. "Why are you saying this? It will work out. If they put you on the list then that's what we'll do, and you'll get better."

Jackie was 100 percent positive about my health condition—always. She never varied. She'd listen when I talked about something going wrong and then say, "We'll see what the doctors say. You'll be fine." She was on a straight forward, positive track for me, but I wasn't sure it was a good thing for her. What if things didn't work out? What were we going to do? It seemed to me she wasn't preparing herself. Nonetheless, that's the way she wanted it, and she stuck with that tack, never looking back. In retrospect, I realize now it was her way of dealing with what she was going through. She needed to deal with it her way.

Everything about a lung transplant was so big and difficult to understand at every turn. We talked about the whole situation over and over, probably feeling as if talking would bring solutions. During one discussion, I said to her, "Ok, look, this is how I feel. I need to tell you this. I won't let my health problems wipe us out. It could. We've heard how things have gone from other friends; you know that. I just can't do that. I can't do that to you, and can't do it to Zachera."

"What are you saying?"

"You know if this IPF thing keeps going the way it is and the doctors put me on a donor list...What I'm saying is...if this whole thing blows up and for a million reasons starts to take our complete savings, everything we've worked so hard for...I won't do it...I mean, I could end up in the hospital for months, who knows... in a home, I don't know. It could drain everything we have." I knew I was treading on the opposite side of her positive viewpoint, but felt it was necessary.

"We have insurance," Jackie said flatly.

"Yeah, but...I don't know. Our other friends had insurance, too, and you saw what happened to them in the end. It's not just the surgery, it's all the costs that go with it and after it. You know what I mean. Remember my mom's friend, Dorothy. Her husband got sick and never got better. She spent some of her prime years taking care of him. He was in a wheelchair, couldn't go to the bathroom alone, couldn't feed himself. She had no life. After years of that, she couldn't take it anymore and they got a divorce. I never blamed her. We only get one life and to spend it as a nurse for twenty years is too much. Thank goodness she got remarried. I don't want to even think about that with you. I'm not doing it."

"None of that is going to happen. You know I'll be here no matter what happens."

My face dropped. "That's just it. It's not about 'no matter what happens'. It's about what I'm going to do about it. I'm not leaving this up to chance. I'm never going there. I'm not."

She said, "What do you mean?"

"I mean, the way this whole IPF thing and MMHMMM's transplant program is headed, I'm going to have to make a decision."

"A decision? On what hospital to go to? I thought..."

"No, not what hospital. Whether to go ahead with the whole thing, or let it go."

Jackie looked at me with wider eyes. As I said, we hadn't broached this yet, not even close. "I have to make a decision on whether to have a transplant or not."

"There isn't a choice, you know that," she said, looking at me incredulously.

"Actually, there is."

Still backing up, Jackie said, "The doctors said a transplant was the only thing we could do. Why are you talking about a choice?"

Looking straight into her eyes, I said, "There is another choice. What if I don't want to have a transplant? What if it's all too much? What if we lose everything we own, we've saved for...everything... trying to cure my IPF? What if I can't do that?"

"You have to."

"Do I?"

Jackie shifted in her chair and I knew she was getting upset. I was getting upset. She put down her book. I knew she would never say, "What about me?" That wasn't in her. But I knew she would bring up Zachera.

Moving up to the edge of her seat, Jackie said, "You have to fight this. We'll be ok. We have insurance. That will cover a lot of it and if it takes some of our savings, that's what we saved it for—emergencies and things like that. Well...now we have an emergency, and if we need more money, that's what we'll use it for."

"I know how you feel. But that's not how I feel," I said, looking away from her.

Jackie was getting more and more distraught. I knew this would happen because no matter how you stirred the soup, it came out the same. She refused to even broach the subject. I tried another tactic: "It's all up in the air. I don't know where it's taking us. What I do know is, I'm not doing it if it wipes us out. I won't. "

Jackie moved over to my chair and sat with me. She sat there a minute and then put her hand on mine. "We can't talk like this. We have to wait until we have the facts. All the facts. We have no idea what's going to happen, and speculating on cost, our savings, all of it, just doesn't make sense right now. We're meeting with the transplant team a week from Monday. Let's wait to discuss this when more information is on the table—when they tell us everything. We don't know enough to do this now." I turned to Jackie and looked into her beautiful eyes, as I always had. We sat there close for quite a while. Things in life had been serious before, but what we were up against now was different. Prior problems weren't about dying.

11

Lung Transplant Forum

Walking into my first lung transplant forum felt so very odd. It's a gathering of patients that offers them a chance to gain information about their transplant and discuss thoughts, ideas, and concerns with other patients who went through the same experience or are about to. It felt odd because, once again, I never pictured myself taking part in a health forum about anything, let alone my lungs.

I was apprehensive because everything happened so fast. One minute I was living in my small town in northern Michigan and then all of a sudden, I was attending a forum in one of the biggest cities in the U.S. with the title "Caring for Your Transplant Lungs." Should I take notes, say anything, keep quiet? What were the other patients going to be like? Was I walking into a room full of extremely sick people? Would patients add comments and be able to talk, or was this just a presentation? Like everything in the last few months, it was all new.

Jackie and Zachera didn't need to come with me. They wanted to, but all of this was so overwhelming, I said, "I want to go by myself this first time. I need to." I knew they'd argue and for good reason, but it was extremely personal to me.

The way I saw it, lots of really big things were about to happen to me—good or bad—and I was going to have to deal with them myself first. I was going to have to get my head straight about all of it, before everyone else could help me. It had to be me...then all the wonderful people supporting me. It was the "you have to love yourself before you can love another" theory. Deep inside I knew I had to grab my own reins and ride.

To be honest, one of the reasons I didn't want them to attend this forum was because the image I had in my head was that of wheelchairs, people with oxygen tanks, air lines running to their nose, patients sick and dying, tubes everywhere, incessant coughing, monitors beeping, and nurses trying to keep their patients comfortable and somewhat coherent. I was afraid it would scare them. It was already scaring me.

There had been tough times in my life. If things got harsh, I could take it because I had to. What was going to happen was going to be tougher than anything I'd ever been through. No question. It didn't take a genius to figure that out. There wasn't any reason to put my family through it, though. Support time would come for them, but it didn't have to be now. If I wanted to stay alive, things like this were necessary, but not for them...yet.

Jackie said, "I came down to Chicago to be with you during things like this."

I countered with, "I know, but this is one thing I want to do by myself. I don't know, I just want to go and let it all soak in. It's personal. I have no idea what's going to happen. Actually, I have no idea about any of this, so I just want to go alone this first time." Zachera was giving me a disparaging look, but I insisted, "I don't know why, but it's what I want for today, ok? There will be other meetings, forums, from the sound of it." They agreed—this time.

So, I went alone. After figuring out where to park, Paul's instructions through MMHMMM's vast hallways and glassed-in overpasses spanning Chicago's streets below led me to a whole new hospital area called the Women's Center, which included a children's wing as well. I passed bright-colored, plastic ocean creatures which were part of a children's play exhibit with a grotto of smiling fish in mid-air, an octopus with big red lips, and upbeat music. Rounding another corner, I came upon Room J, which was where

Paul sent me. I hesitated, but opened the large door. There were about twenty or twenty-five people chatting with each other. Some were in chairs and some standing about. There were women and men, some older, a few younger. Obviously, the meeting hadn't started. Bottled water was lined up on a counter and I headed in that direction for lack of knowing what else to do.

Paul's forum was not at all what I had expected. Patients were standing about like they were perfectly fine. As I looked around, there was only one wheelchair and the person in it looked healthy and was laughing. Her husband was sitting next to her and seemed upbeat as well. Everyone seemed cheery, not at all morose, down, or pessimistic. It was far from what I expected. I thought people would be downcast and depressed, but I found them excited about a new future, about a time where they wouldn't be strapped to an oxygen machine, a time where they had their lives back. My eyes welled up. What was I doing?

I felt so out of place. My mind was not centered. Ever since Dr. Danzer had me meet the lung transplant team, so much was up in the air, vague, and unimaginable. Everything happened so quickly. Was I really doing this?

A middle-aged man walked up to me and said, "Hi, I'm Bob." He was tall and lanky, with the same grey-white hair as most of the men in the room, other than Paul and some male nurses. He had on jeans, a plaid shirt, and running shoes. I had on a white, long-sleeved button-down shirt and my sports jacket. I was the only man in the room with a sports jacket. Everyone was casual, easygoing, no stress, even down to their clothes. The whole atmosphere was so different than I expected; it threw me.

I finally answered, "My name's Bob, too. Actually, it's Robert, but you know how that is," and shook his hand, as old guys do. No chest bumps. Today it seems you either chest bump or just say "Hi" and do nothing. Handshakes are out evidently, but people still put the ol' paw out there, so you don't know what to do!? Hugging is nice, I guess, but very awkward, especially when I meet a woman I don't know. I'm always relieved when the woman quickly sticks out her hand. Whew! I don't have to do some strange kind of side-bump, kind of forward-dip maneuver. I've noticed some younger people just touch the edge of their shoulders together. What issss that? Is that sort of a half bump? Like bumping, "Hi, but I really don't mean it"? It's weird. I'm not a millennial.

"Alright, Bob, I think I can remember that name. But these days, I'm not so sure!"

I said, "I understand completely!"

Bob said, "Are you here for the lung transplant forum?"

"Yes, I hope I'm in the right place," I said as I looked around for Paul.

"You are. This is the right room, and Paul is over there talking to that couple."

I said, "Paul...ah...yeah, he's the fellow who told me about this group. He told me how to get here and all, which wasn't exactly easy!"

"Yeah, well MMHMMM is so big it's hard to find your way around, especially if you're a pre."

I looked at him confused, "A pre?"

"Pre or post?" he asked.

I wasn't sure if that was a question or what. I was in a fog to begin with, so what he said made no sense. It was like someone walking up and asking, "Are you a cantaloupe?" I tried wading through ideas in my mind and came up with nothing. "Um, I don't know." I was trying not to seem totally clueless. "Are some of these people hospital staff?"

Bob said, laughing, "I know it's a lot to take in when you first enter the program. We've all gone through that. It's very confusing, at first. Well, actually, all the time."

"These are all lung transplant patients?" I asked.

Bob explained, "Just about everyone here is in MMHMMM's lung transplant program except Paul, our clinical psychologist, the nurses, and Dr. Danzer, who's presenting today. He's going to talk to us about medications and side effects. There's usually someone from the lung team presenting information."

"Well, thanks for introducing yourself. I don't know anyone and don't know a thing about any of this. You mentioned something about being a 'pre'?"

"Oh…ah…yes. You're a 'pre' because you're 'pre transplant'. There are only two 'pres' here, you and Ginny over there," he said, pointing to a young, maybe twenty-year-old woman.

"You mean that young woman's a pre-lung-transplant patient?" I said incredulously.

Bob said, "I know. You hate to see someone that young have to be involved in all this. Us older patients have had our day, so to speak, but twenty? So, it's you and her that are 'pre.' The rest of us are 'post'—post-transplant."

"You mean you've had a lung transplant?" I asked in amazement. Up until now I had never really met someone who had actually had one, but here was a fit and healthy-looking man standing in front of me. No tubes, no oxygen tank.

Bob said, "Yes, year out. Got my lungs October 27th, 2014. It's a date you never forget."

"Wow. You had a double-lung transplant?" which was a dumb thing to say, since he'd just told me. I was like comedian Bob Farley saying, "Wow. You're Paul McCartney, aren't you!?" I guess it was more of a statement to get my thoughts straight.

Truly, my world was upside down and everything, including going to a lung transplant forum, was throwing me askew, off-kilter. Everything was a blur, but it was more than that. It was too big of a concept to just accept like, "Oh yeah, so we'll talk about getting a lung transplant and then mosey on over to a Chicago Cubs game." Bob said your actual transplant date is a date you'll never forget.

He was right.

Bob replied, "Yes, I had a double. The team felt I was strong enough to do both lungs. They feel you have a better chance of a healthier life if you can replace both lungs. Of course, it depends on a patient's particular situation. Some patients here today only received one lung and are doing well."

Even though everything was overwhelming, I wanted to know

more. I asked, "Is the operation the same when you receive one vs. two? I mean physically, like the way they do it?"

"No—completely different. They enter from the side when they're doing one lung. It's put in from the side, like here." Bob pointed to a spot beneath his right arm.

Standing there listening to how a lung is put into you, how it is inserted, seemed like an eerie dream. Was I going to suddenly wake up and look out my bedroom window thinking, *Ah...well, that was disturbing.* Would I forget about it and just go about my normal day? This was very odd terrain.

Bob continued, "If you are lucky enough to be able to do both lungs, they open up the front of your chest all the way across, from armpit to armpit, sort of cut you in half. It's called a 'clam shell' surgery." Bob took his finger and ran a line from one side of himself to the other. "Then, they lift up your chest cavity and take both lungs out. Once the bad lungs are out, in go the new ones." After Bob's detailed explanation, I knew not having Jackie or Zachera with me was a good idea. I also knew there was more detail in between Bob's "bad lungs out, new lungs in." Much, much more.

In the middle of this discussion, my head felt like a balloon. This was all too much. I wanted to leave. The gentleman I was talking to sensed my bewildered state and said, "Here, let's get some coffee or a drink and find a seat, ok?"

I've never fainted. I've been knocked out a few times playing sports, but that was different. This felt like something was happening to me inside. I couldn't shake the feeling. It was as if I was in some far-off movie and wanted it to stop so I could step out of the frame. But, I couldn't. I stood there motionless.

Thoughts raced through my head. I can't be doing this. This is going to change my life as I know it. One of those patients is in a wheelchair. I can't do that. I won't be able to drive our car, fix things around the house, shovel the driveway during the snowy months up north. Bob said, "they sort of cut you in half." How can anyone live through that? How can they do that? What about Jackie. What about her life? She can't spend the rest of our days taking care of me, wheeling me around, doing everything for me. I don't want Zachera and Ryan to do this. What about our savings? I'm not losing everything Jackie and I saved while teaching for forty years. It wasn't much on a teacher's salary, but it was money we saved to make sure Jackie would be ok if something happened to me. We wanted Zachera and Ryan to have something from us when we were gone. We worked hard and it was difficult to save. I'm not doing this. Maybe I'll be ok. Maybe the tests showing I need a lung transplant are false readings. I can work things out—I can get out of this. I couldn't stop my mind from repeating it over and over: *I can get out of this...I can get out of this.*

"You want water, Pepsi, or a coffee?" Bob said, jarring me back into the forum.

In a stupor, I said, "Ah, yeah...um...I'll take a Pepsi, thanks."

With Paul's directions in my hand, Bob and I landed in two chairs making up part of a large circle of patients, their family members and friends, and Paul. Nurses took a seat behind patients they were attending. Everyone began to sit down. Next to me was an older man with grey hair and a pony tail. He looked like a bigger, younger Willie Nelson. Well, I mean, everyone looks younger than Willie Nelson. He was friendly and introduced himself. His name was John.

The people in the room—now seated—were a mix of males and females of all different ages. It looked like a United Nations meeting because there were different ethnicities, clothes, and dialects, something I wasn't used to living in rural northern Michigan. It was like back in my days growing up in Detroit.

Some men had on sweaters, some just casual shirts and jeans. The women in the group wore different outfits, from dresses to jeans and blouses. About half the group had medical masks on, the muddy yellow kind—which always looked to me like a sort of urine yellow. I've seen blue ones around, but only on staff members. Who came up with that ugly yellow? Having to wear one was bad enough, so, by all means, let's make it pukey looking? Others in the room didn't have masks on. They didn't seem too concerned about germs or contracting anything from the others. I wondered why some did, some didn't?

Paul brought the meeting to order, so to speak. Not in a formal way; he was more relaxed and friendly. What struck me immediately was how professionally Paul handled everything. He started off with the group's policy regarding how to deal with personal information and thoughts and ideas shared in the group. We needed to keep all information in the room. Other than general information like first names, etc., personal thoughts in the forum were not to be made public. Asking someone what happened in terms of their health, their surgery, was not allowed. If someone wanted to tell you or the group about their experience, that was fine. But it was their choice. Asking someone what was wrong or which operation they went through breached their privacy. Paul mentioned it was important to be courteous and not dominate the discussion, and to give everyone a chance to speak.

Paul was very calm. He set the meeting's tone by taking his time, explaining things thoroughly, and making everyone feel comfortable. He was dark-haired and surprisingly young, maybe thirty-five years old. He was slender, about six feet two in height, and wore a dark button-down shirt with casual pants, which was different than doctors I had seen so far. They all had long white doctor coats with their name embroidered in navy blue below their right lapel. Most of the male doctors wore a tie; female doctors seemed to wear buttoned-up blouses with some sort of necklace or pendant. Every move Paul made, what he wore, his demeanor, body language, and mild voice, had a theme: calm and non-threatening.

It was immediately apparent Paul viewed us as more than patients, more like friends. It was a feeling he exuded. It was clear he cared about everyone in the room. As it turned out, I never spent a moment with Paul where he wasn't attentive and caring. He seemed like a person who had found the perfect job for his personality—a vocation.

At first, Paul's rules seemed over-the-top for just a small group of people discussing things, but this forum was far more important than expected, and no ordinary group. They were incredibly strong. Taking part ended up being one of the top healing forces for my mental state.

Most of the time, a MMHMMM staff person would present information on things like the proper diet for a transplant patient—don't eat mushrooms, blue cheese, etc. —or how to exercise or shower without tearing incisions, things of that nature. If a doctor or specialist couldn't make the forum, Paul would run it. He would start with a general topic relating to our situation and then let us give our thoughts.

Dr. Danzer was delayed in the hospital, so Paul said, "Since it's going to be a few moments before Dr. Danzer can get here, let's talk about events and things that were difficult for you to deal with after your surgery."

Immediately, an older black woman, who might have weighed ninety-five pounds, maybe, raised her hand. "Hello, everyone, I'm Marta Rae, and I think havin' all this incontinence thing is a major pain in the ass."

I was really surprised by this woman's open thoughts on what usually is a pretty private subject. But then I became impressed by a number of things. One: this woman had some sass. I loved it. She didn't beat around the bush. Two: who would have guessed this strong personality would come from such a small, demure person? Three: she went on to explain—exactly—no holds barred—what happened to her each day in terms of going to the bathroom and how damn pissed off—no pun intended—she was her doctors couldn't fix it. She added she loved her doctors, but was mad at the moment because they weren't "takin' care of bidness fixin' her down below."

Quite an introduction to the forum! Evidently, this was the real deal, a place where you could say what was on your mind, where you could bring up any topic you needed to talk about. Informing from the git-go.

The topic of incontinence got everyone involved right away. Obviously, it was a common problem. Many talked about how they handled it, remedies, what worked best, situations they had gone through, and how to avoid them. What an interesting group. This forum was far different than pictured. I imagined bleak patients, some on gurneys, with foggy mental states from heavy drugs. The fact that I didn't know a damn thing about any of it was to blame. I was wayyyy off. This was one serious, informed, and tough group.

Paul helped by clarifying medical procedures when needed, moved things forward when someone got a bit off track, and nudged, for lack of a better word, shy patients to enter the conversation. He quietly watched each person as patients spoke to see if someone wanted to say something but didn't want to interrupt. He'd come back to them when there was a pause and say, "Ginny, it looked like you had something to say about...?" and Ginny would then add her thoughts. She seemed like a very quiet person; if he hadn't noticed her, she wouldn't have spoken up.

The patients' stories were incredible. What massively resilient individuals. How did they survive? Some came through their transplant fairly well, some didn't. One fairly young woman said she had been in the hospital for five straight months and had just gotten out. Everyone applauded and she seemed to really appreciate their support. My mind couldn't comprehend being in a hospital for so long. How did she make it through? Shots, procedures, tests, how her list must have run on and on.

These were people from all walks of life: construction workers, teachers, firemen, accountants. They came from different areas around the country, from small towns to large cities like Chicago. Other than the two "pres," Ginny and evidently me, each person had undergone a huge, immensely dangerous surgery and there they were sitting next to me, completely normal. I knew they weren't; they couldn't be, but they sure seemed happy and full of life.

There were couples sitting next to each other. Tough issues or not, I shouldn't have discouraged Jackie to come. She probably needed to hear what the group had to say, but I was in protective mode and didn't want her to get hurt or scared. So much laid in front of us. I had no idea what this forum was going to be like. What if they talked about gruesome details that went wrong, about patients dying? I thought it might be unsettling and felt the same regarding Zachera. Why put both of them through all of this?

On the other hand, maybe the reality that they were now part of the whole program whether they wanted to be or not needed to be out in the open. I couldn't buffer them; it was happening—a storm I couldn't hold back. We were all in this.

Thoughts ran through my head. All of a sudden, Paul asked me if I could tell the group who I was and what I was thinking about since I was a "pre." I stuttered, not expecting to talk, "Ah...ah... well...this is all so much...you know. Ah..." Some patients nodded their heads, as if saying, "I've been there." I stammered on, "I... ah...well...my name is Robert, and..." Not knowing whether it was appropriate or not, I said, "I might...um...according to the team, need new lungs."

Actually, I didn't know what to say. To me, that was it. Being there summed it up. It was all so new and mind blowing, to use a cliché. Paul helped by asking, "What led you to MMHMMM?"

"Ah...My daughter, actually...Um...I was coughing a lot, and... my wife Jackie kept asking me to get it checked out, and...then my daughter started pleading with me to come to MMHMMM to... you know, see what was going on." Again, the patients seemed to know. They'd gone through the same thing.

Paul stepped in, "Did anyone here have that happen to them?"

Immediately, hands were raised and many spoke about being scared, not wanting to find out results, ignoring danger signs, being embarrassed, worried about their family, worried about what might happen to them. Some brought up the word "denial," which hit home.

Paul's forum turned out to be informative and emotional. Throughout my time at MMHMMM and afterwards, Paul's forums provided a tremendous amount of help and encouragement. Sitting and talking with twenty or so people who went through the same situations, the same difficult tasks, the same dark moments, meant so much to me. Somehow, I felt safe and strong at the same time being with them. I can't explain it. Groups made up of people from similar backgrounds and common—or, in this case, very uncommon— experiences hold a unified sort of power when they're together.

A while back, I spent some time with World War II vets in the same kind of forum, the bond was the same. They had gone through unspeakable moments and nodded the same way when someone spoke. Nodded because they had been there, nodded because they knew. From my very first day attending Paul's forum, I felt stronger. These patients got through it, they weathered the storm, and were sailing again. They had their bodies ravished and were now strong. How incredible is that. They had someone else's lungs put in their chest, and they were living and laughing. How awe-inspiring it was to be with them.

Chicago is a long way from where I live, but I try to schedule my clinic—which is a recurring three- or four-month lung checkup—in the same week as Paul's forums. They take place once a month on Wednesdays. Something new is always covered, and attending and reveling with such a brave and fierce group makes me feel resilient.

It was during one of Paul's forums I finally let myself accept what was going to happen. Until that point, a lung transplant was something that happened to other people. My lungs were deteriorating, but I just couldn't go there. I had to get my thoughts straight, to resolve—in my own mind—a head-on approach to it all. Sitting next to human beings who had faced the same darkness—that they soon might die—suddenly hit home all at once. They did it. How, I didn't know, but here they were. The old adage "If they can do it, I can too" became perfectly clear. More importantly, I finally had something to end my denial and start my journey forward.

12

Resolve

In the following days , my emotions flowed and somewhat settled down to a dull WTF. Thanks to my lung transplant team and Paul's forums, I was able to confront what was ahead of me. An understanding, which was another part of the process, another piece of the puzzle, took place. As it turned out, it was one of the most important pieces to my successful double-lung transplant. It's difficult to write about because it's conceptual, not something black-and-white pinpointed on a graph or a lit x-ray screen. So many people are curious about the lung transplant details, percentages, numbers. They want to know how long you might live, how long a donor lung will last, what meds you're taking, how many pills a day. But, as it surprisingly turned out, there is an overriding umbrella over everything—a powerful force we have inside us.

Many medical studies show a strong correlation between a patient's conceptual belief and their physical being. What you visualize, what you truly believe, can morph into your physical being. I know it can. It did for me. Resolve came to me like a freight train.

I lived through my double-lung transplant. Recovery, which will always be ongoing, happened—I truly believe—because of a moment of resolve. After learning what a lung transplant was all about, reading, talking with doctors, doing what I could to understand, meeting with the lung transplant team, long discussions with my family, and hours of private thought, I decided to flat-out do it.

I resolved to use every ounce of strength I had in my body to make it through…and live. A decision that outwardly seemed simple, but was deeply complicated.

Resolve is defined as coming *to a definite or earnest decision about* something. Please understand the word "resolve" is synonymous with words like power, strength, courage, bravery, commitment, determination, toughness, and tenacity. It had to be because of what I was going to undergo. My chances of survival were in a different category than most. Imagine for a few minutes what would it be like if a doctor told you your surgery was extremely difficult and you may not make it through. What do you think would go through your mind? How would you handle it? To survive, at some point you would need to build answers to those questions. Heading into something that intense without a solid, set resolve would be disastrous. I can't imagine how scary that would be. I knew I had to answer my own questions.

Heavy, heavy questions sat across the table from me. I had to face them. But, when it got right down to it, to the very base level, there was truly only one over-riding question, and just one answer. For me, giving up and dying was not an option. Can you do it? To resolve to get through everything—no matter what—was the only answer.

Giving up did not exist. Going into such an incredibly complicated surgery being scared and saddled with trepidation didn't make sense either. It was all or nothing, in my mind.

At some point, on that particular day, and after learning as much as possible about what was going to happen to me, I had a heart-to-heart talk with myself, cliché aside. It was a must; it had to happen. It was a moment. A special moment.

I took my time. After sitting quietly, I resolved to live for myself, my family, and my friends. I remember it was a distinctly physical thing…as if it existed right in front of me, as if I could touch it. Real…because it was, 100 percent. No grey area. It was one of the strongest feelings I've ever had, and I expect it was a feeling, a commitment, many others in my lung transplant program had as well. How could they have survived without it?

Please understand, there are many, many different components to a double-lung transplant, to say the least. I don't want to imply that coming to a personal resolve makes everything fine and rosy. It's just that I believe it was the most important aspect for my personal survival. Everyone is different. Depending on the circumstances, other components might be as important or even more so. There's no set roadmap, no exact rules. The truth is, a donor family, my doctors, and my lung transplant team saved me. My resolve saved me, as well.

When someone asks me what the most important element in my successful transplant experience was, the answer is twofold: my lung team, and my resolve. We all look at life differently and handle things the best way we can. That's it. We do what we can. No script.

The sidekick of resolve is intent. Intent is also incredibly important in terms of a mindset towards a goal and eventually achieving it. Intent is defined as directing one's mind or energy to committing to a plan.

It's imperative to bring these concepts up because they answer the question "What's the one thing you did to get through it all?" Whether this sounds like an infomercial for My Pillow, deep inside having resolve and intent in my mind and heart before heading into the most crucial moment of my life simply gave me a personal power.

After I survived my transplant, Zachera and Ryan gave me a t-shirt with a picture of lungs on the front. Above the lungs it read, "I survived a double-lung transplant." Below the lungs, it finished with, "What's your Super Power?" Each and every lung transplant patient I met had a super power. Resolve makes you strong. I'll say it over and over: the lung transplant survivors I spent time with at MMHMMM were the strongest people I've ever met.

In case you are thinking I'm an intensely disciplined person to get through what transplant patients endure, a disciplined person I—am—not! Far from it. Making and breaking rules throughout my life has been sort of a hobby. Life wouldn't be fun running in a straight line all the time. I mean, I've tried to keep this habit to a minimum because said mode can cost you money—parking tickets (I think I broke the MSU record for student parking tickets received in one semester), speeding tickets, U-turns, you name it. I actually got a ticket for jaywalking once. Not kidding. (Not sure younger people even know that term.) Then, there's the "trying to lose weight and then bingeing on Lafayette Coney dogs with mustard, no onion, and a side of large fries," like we do. Deciding it would be cool to run the Detroit Marathon with no disciplined yearlong training program just about ruined my body (the "please don't try this at home" thing). Even so, I made it to the finish line and will never forget it. Tried the fiddle, learned two songs, done. Different instruments, nope. (I now have an arsenal of unconquered musical instruments.) The list goes on. When it comes to human beans and discipline, tough match. It's a struggle for me.

I'm only telling you this to make an important point: making such a strong commitment to get through my upcoming transplant ordeal saved me. No doubt. One hundred percent resolve. That's it. I'm doing this, no matter what.

There were days where my resolve was tested, and tested severely, and each time, I said to myself over and over, "I will not give in." I repeated this to myself each day like a mantra. No one knew. I did it privately because I felt telling someone might take away some of my intent's power. It had to be a private resolve because I knew intrinsically I was the only one who could make it really happen. Everyone around you will try to help, but deep inside, it's you. It has to be you and no one else. People helped me at every turn, but, ultimately, it came down to whether or not I wanted to stay alive.

Writing about my resolve was an incredibly important part of this book because my main goal was to help others going through similar life-changing experiences. Yes, it was my personal resolve, but it was too powerful to leave out. When I'm together with "pre" lung patients, they tell me what they're thinking and what they want to know. Invariably they ask, "How did you get through it? How am I going to get through it?" My answer is the same each time, "I resolved in my own mind to never quit, to give it my all no matter what, and, if I did that, whether I lived or not, at least I tried." It was that big. It saved me.

For the first time in my crazy life, I stuck to my plan. There were days I didn't do as well as I could have—the discipline thing showed up—but I tried. Before my transplant, it was difficult to lose the weight my doctors required. I had a bad day here and there, but I never broke my personal promise. I never will. Eventually, at some moment, I'll die, but as Dylan Thomas says, I'll "never go gently into the night."

Why? I thought about it a lot. Considerations roll around in your head when you face the reality of your situation. There are many different paths to take when something in life is threatening, but the question "Why?" kept showing up on the top of the list. I had to answer it to move on. If I didn't answer, I knew I'd never get to my base level, the bottom line. I'd never get to where I had to be.

To me, getting to the root—or base—of why you're living and how you personally feel about it is central. Maybe many people are frightened when something severe happens because they've never truly touched their base, their reason for living. I don't know. I'm not a psychologist. But what I do know is, when confronted with the fact that I might die soon, I had to come to grips with it right away. Like Emeril would yell, "Bam!" right now, I had to. To put it off, to not answer, would leave my mind in a terrible state of flux. If the end came, my mind wouldn't be where it needed to be.

Whether I wanted to or not, dealing with dying had to be head-on. If I could firmly decide how I felt, what I believed, I'd be ok. So, I did and never looked back. There's a life energy in all of us. I can feel it. I felt it leaving me as I started to drown in the waters of Lake Charlevoix. When I was born, my mother gave it to me. Why in the world let it go? Why not fight to stay alive as long as I had a quality of life for myself and my family? I was given energy to live, not to let it float slowly away on a Viking funeral pyre.

There's a massive difference between fighting to stay alive and ending life when it's truly over. If I have a quality of life worth living, I'll fight to the end. I'll be the warrior and never give up. If I don't have a quality of life, it will be, as Maude said in the famous movie *Harold and Maude*, "time to move on to a new adventure."

Everyone's different. I have no idea whether the above resolve approach will work for someone else. It's what I confronted in my mind and where I went. I survived. Having such a brilliant, positive partner like Jackie helped get my mind straight when I needed to.

MMHMMM's lung transplant team continually brought up strong family and close friends. The team knew the strength such support groups provide. Zachera and Ryan gave me needed care, whether it entailed camping at their house, cooking dinners, rides to the hospital, trying to get my mind off my situation, or caring for me in any way they could. For them, it was the "whatever it takes," the "no matter what" attitude. I love them for that.

There's power in the phrase "no matter what." It speaks volumes. It's not a lightweight phrase. Think about it. "I'll never give up—no matter what," and "I'll always love you—no matter what." Powerful personal statements that exemplify major resolve when you need it the most.

When a pre-lung-transplant patient asks, "What's the most important thing I can do before going ahead with a transplant?" my answer is always the same. "Resolve your own commitment and never give it up."

"No matter what."

13

The Twilight Zone

I strongly suggest getting a glass of wine or a beer, a shot, a Vernors (if you're from Detroit), maybe with something in it, right now.

Alright, if you've done the resolve thing and your head is secure, you need to read this because you can now handle it.

So, there I was heading into the testing phase of getting a lung transplant to see if my body qualified to get on the list. Did I believe they would go through my whole goddamn body and notttt find something wrong here or there—no. But I was willing to try. Resolve. Well…the giving up was no option idea showed up again. Just keeps workin' in there, I don't know. Testing took weeks and weeks.

The national organ donor organization only gives organs to healthy patients, which seems to make no sense. But when you break it down, what that really means is, patients who are healthy enough to withstand a transplant. Healthy besides a specific problem. In my case, lungs. They had to make sure the rest of me was A-OK. You wouldn't buy a used car if you didn't have it checked out, right? I was now at the hospital's equivalent of Car Max.

The donor organization needs solid factual reasons to believe you are under seventy years old, fairly ok, only fart occasionally, and won't die during surgery. Sorry, but it's that kind of deal. National donor recipients must be fairly strong—give or take—and in somewhat decent physical condition. It's obvious why. Also sad because, unfortunately, there are more people needing transplants than there are donors each year. We need more donors. It's one of the reasons I'm writing this book.

Once put on the Disney Pass Every Test Imaginable Matterhorn Thrill Ride, I was suddenly a common name on the myriad of doctor lists involving what I call "checking out my stuff." If you're heading into a transplant of any kind, major surgery, or putt-putt golf, read this. If you're heading into a bar, read this tomorrow.

So, this chapter is a heads-up, a "hey, you need to know this." It's also an answer for patients who ask after they go through some type of adversity, "Why in the hell didn't someone tell me about all this ahead of time!!?!?" If we ever meet on the street or at a party, you can shake my hand and thank me for informing you. Maybe you'll say you didn't like all the swearing, but how else could I convey all this damn stuff! I think I warned you—maybe not. Yes, I did warn you!

In retrospect, I should've known about all this hospital para-phernalia before ending up smack dab in the middle of it. But, as Paul, my guiding light, said so profoundly, "We need a book about transplants from a patient's perspective." If for no other reason, read all the pages so you won't be "spidered" (see chapter 3 1/2). If you're not getting a transplant, the following is a glimpse into a very bizarre world. I mean, you watch all this on Netflix or Prime, so why not delve into the real deal?

If you're not doing well health-wise and are headed into some type of hospital procedure, this chapter will be pertinent. When your friends say, "You told me about some lung book. What's it about?" you can truthfully tell them, "Science fiction." Sorry, but that's what a transplant or any other serious surgery is. Strange science fiction, Dr. Strangelove stuff, but actually what doctors, nurses, and hospitals do every day.

Truly, once you enter this Zone, you will be one with the strang-est names you've never heard of. You'll meet up with wild-look-ing instruments, futuristic rooms, people with no faces (masks), bedpans, tubes going in, tubes going out, buckets (if buckets are involved, it's not good), acronyms flowing like another language, smells (which will get its own chapter) hand sanitizer absolutely everywhere, people walking up suddenly and saying, "Sanitizer!" your own urine-yellow face mask (who in the hell picked that color?), aluminum walking rigs with wheels, hooks for your buckets, bags, shit, urine, weird-colored fluids, a magazine rack, Starbucks holders, directions, and WiFi. Railings everywhere to make sure you stay upright.

People will stroll by saying, "Whoa, I hope I don't get what he has," and my all-time favorite: frozen soup. Science fiction?! Here's one. We take lunch for granted. One fun day, a day nurse named Sheshawnna delivered my hospital lunch. I really had no idea what her real name was, but that's what I heard her say to another staff member. MMHMMM is about as downtown Chicago as you can get, and, because of that, they have a very diverse workforce. "Ship"—her nickname—came from Ghana. I loved talking to all the different staff members, asking about the areas of Chicago where they lived, and where they were from originally. It gave me something interesting to do while looking at my blank beige hospital walls.

The soup thing happened when Sheshawnna set a light-brown, food-court plastic tray down on my nifty rolling tray stand. Nothing makes food look better than a brown/beige/puke-colored tray. Couldn't someone come in one night and spray-paint all of those trays blue or something fun? Of course, once said tray is placed next to your bed, whomever brought it leaves. Then, when you touch it, your stand rolls justttt out of reach. You lean out and try to catch it, but farther and farther away from your bed it goes. One time it went in the next room. It was possessed. My grilled cheese got cold.

My lunch tray usually contained a semi-strange, midday meal some orderly delivered. Sheshawnna started doing whatever job nurses do around the room, and I decided to try my spiffy lunch. The sandwich wasn't all bad: fairly dry bread, old tuna something, probably some mayo in there somewhere, and a sprig of dried-up limp parsley. Why do they include items like that? It's not like old limp parsley adds to the ambience. Probably some kitchen vice-semi-manager made a massive decision, "Add some parsley to make the meals look better." To which one of the orderlies said under her breath, "Puttin' dead parsley on dat shit ain't helpin'." Not to mention having something "limp" around doesn't help males' egos.

After not being impressed by the first sandwich bite, I looked around on the tray for something I might semi-enjoy. As I started peeling the plastic top off the rubbery tub holding soup, I thought, "You can't mess up soup," a counter to the balsa-wood bread. The container was oddly cold. *Hmmm, French Vichyssoise?* At a hospital? Nope.

Frozen soup.

I looked up at Sheshawnna, who was hooking up some weird machine at the bottom of my bed and said, "Ship, this is just crazy."

From below the bed I heard, "Get used to it, hon. All thangs crazy roun' here."

"I know, but...ah...I don't think this soup is going to work."

Ship slowly got up, swearing under her breath, rubbed her knees, and gave me the nurse stare. The one where they look at you blankly and don't say anything. Finally, she offered a tired, disgruntled health tip, "Don't give me no guffer, mon, eat da soup. Soup good for you."

I said, "Yeah, but it's frozen."

I didn't add "fucking" before "frozen" because you have to be really nice to nurses. They may or may not respond quickly when you urgently hit the call button because you urgently have to go to the bathroom. You get the picture. There's a whole list of needs and wants nurses provide, so it was imperative I stayed on her good side. I had to tread lightly—Ship was moody.

She moved menacingly closer. "Wat you say 'bout soup?"

"Ahhh, the soup...it's...ah...frozen."

Ship immediately stuck her finger into the ice-crusted soup, which made me laugh.

"I'll be damned. Soup be frozen! Shit. I'm givin that kitchen the what-be-do. No damn reason for it, no reason at all," she said as she grabbed my tray and headed out the door to do what she called "some ass whippin'."

I loved my nurses—female and male. They did great work. If they didn't, they at least tried hard. Actually, many funny things happened surrounding difficult moments with me, but let me say for the record, I'm not belittling or downplaying anyone's ordeal by calling it funny. You need to know that levity at difficult moments was one of the reasons I was able to get through it all. Every staff member took matters seriously to a fault. Their business isn't about silly floor review grades. Many times, it has to do with life or death. The difficult work medical workers do day in and day out is tough and demanding. They deserve miles of credit.

With that said, let's move on to the infamous Wacky Language of the Medical World. I truly believe Disney could build a movie around all of it. If not a movie, at least a ride at Disney World where you move along on a gurney and get bombarded with medical acronyms in bright neon colors, with runaway trays, and get slapped with rubber tubes.

You can try to stay with the staff regarding acronyms, even ask questions, but you'll forget the answer about a minute later because of your meds. "Excuse me, but what did you call that prong?" Doesn't matter because they already did what it does. The pace is quick, they move fast. Basically, "Forgetttt aboutttt itttt!"

The whole medical-acronym jargon thing is by design so you don't know what they mean. I mean, you have to understand how much staff time would be sucked up if every patient got a complete and serious explanation of how they separate different parts of your bowel movement in a centrifuge. Even if they did take the time, you wouldn't understand anyway. They know that. After the first few days, just let acronyms zip right over your head. Here's an example:

Nurse walks in my room with her thin outfit wafting about her. She's all business, even though she looks like the fairy godmother's medical assistant. Her body is covered from head to toe in blue, including her shower cap, gown, and puffy-looking booties. The works. She's even got goggles on—blue, of course.

Goggles can't be good. Think about it. Why do they need goggles? What would they be doing that necessitated goggles? Woodcutters use goggles, welders wear metal goggles, sometimes dentists wear goggles. So, I'm feeling uneasy about the whole attire. It's like I've been smeared with some kind of uranium cream stuff whilst being under, and fluffy nurse is going to run a Geiger counter across my body. Crackle, crackle, bizzzz. At that juncture, she takes out all sorts of tools. Never relax if they have tools.

I mean, you really don't know what they do to you when you're under. They could use your stomach as a lunch table; how would you know? You could be completely naked with this plastic tray lying on your not-so-appetizing parts. Jimmy says, "Harry, pass the salt. It's in his belly button."

Harry answers, "Nope, we got fries today. Using his belly button for ketchup."

Maybe it's the major drugs you're on—maybe not.

By the way, if you think I'm making this shit up, try walking through a hospital nuclear lab. You'll come out glowing. "Do they really have something like that?" you ask? Answer: "Yes, they do."

Hospital employees actually go to lunch wearing those blue flowy outfits. Some even keep those stylish blue shower caps on their head whilst eating greasy pizza in the hospital-commons food court. They sit with staff who are also wearing those shower caps. It's weird seeing them in a group of six or seven, with blue Jiffy Pop caps, eating, chatting, and flirting, like balloons bobbing at a county fair. Maybe it's just me, but would some female think you're attractive with your puffy on and a piece of pizza spinach stuck in your teeth?

For the record, there are a lotttt of good-looking women and men in hospital food courts. Most look like students who just graduated from either pre-med or even more impressive, vet school—all talking one hundred mph in excited voices. They have nowhere else to go for lunch because staff breaks are too short. But if I was a young, handsome "Big Swingin' Dick," as they say...I'd sure as hell take off the blue bonnet, which used to be margarine in its day. So, stuff the shower cap in your pocket, bring a different shirt, change in the elevator, and at least try to appear spiffy. I don't know, is it me, or Memorex?

BTW—Who are the "they" in "as they say"? People have been saying that for years, but nobody knows.

Looking at the blue gown / puff cap / booties outfit from another viewpoint, "Big Swingin'" might wear his staff ensemble so people know he's one of them. Hmmm...I may be on to something. A red badge of courage sort of thing. If you came to the food court dressed nice and casual, others might think, "Who the hell is this guy?" or "Yuck, a sick patient," and move to another table. Safety in numbers, commonality, the flock, the gang, ring, clique, posse—I don't know.

Back to wacky medical stuff examples: an older, gruff-looking nurse walked into my room with her fun blue outfit. I said, "Hello!" in a welcoming, cheery voice because peach cobbler was a lunch "pick." Nurse Ratchet's look-a-like moved closer to my bed and staunchly announced, "Here for your IBA."

"Oh, well, ahhhh...okkkk," not knowing what the hell an IBA was.

She takes something out of her tool bag / torture kit and says, "Roll over."

I sit straight up, "Wait. Whoa...Hold up! Roll over? Whatttt are we doing?"

"An IBA."

"Oh, yeah. What was I thinking? The ol' IBA. Yep, sure, I know what that is. Go right ahead and stick that prong up my ass, because if anyone needs an IBA, I sure do! What the hell is an IBA!@!!?"

Making a smirky face, she says, "Relax, sugar, it's just an internattleotosis bottletimemeter ananloguie." Sarcastically I say, "Now I feel better."

So that's how it goes—constantly: some fun stuff, some not-so-fun, some good, some bad, some downright frightening. While stuck in a hospital bed with nothing to do and for your reading/viewing pleasure, I've created a handy dandy info list to help you wade through your medical maze. This is what I found:

IV

IV can be green plants growing on a wall, but probably means, for some reason, sticking you over and over with a needle until they find justttt the right vein. You can watch them do it, but I think staring makes the phlebotomist (blood-drawing gal/guy) nervous. Quite a job. Sticking humans with needles all day. When they stick or administer whatever, I don't like to watch. I stare out in space. My favorite part is when red stuff is running into the plastic vial because that means they're in. They have all sorts of colored vials—green, yellow, and, surprisingly, red. It's tricky work, though.

Here's why. This whole sticking you with a prong/needle/pin/tube doesn't always go smoothly. Two nurses tried to find a specific vein one morning when I was having yet another test. When the procedure started going south, one nurse said, "You've got spider veins."

"Good to know, good to know. What the hell does that mean?" I inquired.

"Some patients have smaller, thin little veins that are hard to find. That's what yours are like. Spider web stuff." The nurse proceeded to prod and poke my arm with no success, and then said to the other, "Let's try up by his shoulder."

Seemed logical. Forearm, hand, upper arm—why not? They rubbed the proverbial alcohol on a patch of my shoulder and actually did find something with blood in it. They pulled off the giant rubber band around my arm, said I'd be fine, and left me in the room with the IV sticking out sideways up by my shoulder. Pretty soon—but not that soon—the doctor, who was going to do some strange thing using the IV, showed up and exclaimed to his assistant, "Why in the hell is this IV sticking out from this patient's shoulder?" He seemed very agitated, which got his assistant agitated, which got me ... worried.

"Yeah, I was wondering the same thing." I would have said "same damn thing," but never piss off doctors with latex gloves. (Rule 52).

IVs can go well, poorly, or be a pain in the ass. You can't live with 'em, you can't live without 'em. I copped this attitude—using an old '50s/'60s term like "copped" for effect—"Gonna happen, gotta happen, so be it." It didn't help, but gave me something to think about whilst they were pricking me all over the place.

"Copped," by the way, was a word thrown around a lot back in the day. Ok, '60s. It showed up most whilst describing to our horny, middle-school friends what we did during Saturday's movie matinée. Shadowy theatre, cute girls, dark aisles, I won't go into detail, but, if you're older you probably catch my drift. "Copped" definitely has a different meaning now. BTW—middle-school girls did this too!

There were IVs wherever I went. If I went down to the bookstore, there was a nurse waiting to give me an IV. They come with the territory. Want lunch? Get an IV. Here's what I found out during the testing section of my stay at MMHMMM:

ASAP

Forget this acronym. It only translates to "hospital time," not real time. ASAP doesn't happen—too busy for ASAP. It's...probably... perchance...maybe...yesterday...tomorrow...sometime...maybe not ...could be. This acronym is used when the staff needs to move you from one room to another or to a spooky place called a procedure room. Don't hold your breath (sorry, lung transplant joke). Gather up something juicy to read, get out your Rubik's Cube, dial up Angry Birds on your cell; it's going to be a long wait. When the physical footprint of your hospital makes up 50 percent of Chicago, you're talkin' a long wait.

SOB

You were probably shocked when you heard a nurse say, "That

patient is an SOB." Wow! Harsh! But, it's not what you're thinking. SOB stands for "shortness of breath." Learn to ignore nurse talk when it's not directed at you. Most of the time, it won't make sense and will get you in trouble.

CDB

Not a bank or money market. Not something you play videos on. Also, not hemp. CDB is a procedure nurses make you do after surgery. It stands for "cough, deep breath" and is done to make sure your pipes aren't clogged with old carburetor fluid. If you cough and a big glob of something flies out, it's good they did it.

Catheter

I know, I know, it's not an acronym, but *this* was the one word, procedure, route, gadget I worried about the most. You might think, why would just one word bother me thatttt much? Holy shit!! Because it has something to do with my penis, that's why! Sacred place, guarded. Athletic stores sell secret-service protective gear for this singular place. "You being taken down for your catheter, Mr. Emmet." Dreaded words, nightmares.

When really scary stuff was coming up, I had to get my head straight to bravely brace for whatever weird procedure was ahead. But, a catheter? Some torture mechanism they used in 900 AD? "Aaarrrr, we'll use the catheter on 'em, then he'll talk!" People always make it out as ten times worse than childbirth. Believe me, I imagined the worst—double worst—which sounds like a sandwich. Prior to my lung transplant, a catheter might have been number three on my all-time list of Things I Never Want to Do In Life. Number one, and a very strong number one, was: holding a tarantula in my hand. Number two: having a young female candy striper, somewhere between sixteen and seventeen years old, give me an enema while I'm completely nude, blown up like a balloon, and haven't had a bowel movement for a week. (And, BTW, it's "striper," not "stripper"—big difference).

People will also tell you tales about how big their catheter needle/probe was. They'd say, "Make sure you ask for the narrow one." Well, no shit, Sherlock!! But, then, as things go in life, the actual procedure didn't hurt at all! Not kidding. Why I was on major drugs...in Never Never Land!! I was so out of it the nurses could have done anything they wanted to me. When I woke up, I semi-remember asking the nurse, "Ah, excuse me, but there seems to be a strange coiled tube coming out from between my legs?" The nurse just smiled and said the now infamous nurse response, "Yep."

There were lots of catheters during my stay. Kudos go to my penis. I mean, it still works and has fun after all that mishandling. It wasn't really mishandling, per se. It was more like a tire rotation. I don't know. In retrospect, my whole body deserves an Oscar for hanging in there and acting like it was fine. It wasn't fine, but, again, how the hell would I know?! Meds!

Here's another thing. People come in your hospital room and actually say, "How ya doin'?" They do! You can come back with, "Well, pilgrim, I'm steady as a horse and tough as leather." Alright, no John Wayne impressions, but what are you supposed to say to a question like that?

Sometimes, they even sit on the edge of your bed, which is nice, but dangerous. One time when visiting my dad in the hospital, I sat on the edge of his bed and the damn thing folded up in a V. Up it went! He was ok after they cranked his bed back down, but I felt like Webster's definition of an idiot. It wasn't my fault; I didn't do anything, but everyone was staring at me like, "He just went through prostate surgery!!"

Here's the deal: don't ask a patient "How ya doin'?" because you're liable to get a response like Robert DeNiro in *Taxi*, "Ya talkin' ta me? Ya talkin' ta me?" Or, "How'm I doin'?! Terrible! Tubes up every orifice, legs like balloons, and I'm taking one in a bedpan at this very minute! That's how I'm doin'!!"

Just a word of warning.

PA

When they talk about "your PA," they are not referring to your long-lost father or a public announcement system. Your PA is your physician's assistant. Become major friends because your PA is very powerful. Do not cross this person. They hold all the strings. Make sure your PA knows any move you make, including movements. They get very upset when you decide to pull tubes out of places on your body, skip meds, or walk around the halls naked, which you'll do because of your meds.

Don't try to get away with shit. Eating jalapeno beef jerky just before surgery, taking gross pictures of your incision and posting it on Facebook, yanking on rubber tubes when you don't know what they're attached to, and everyone's favorite, trying to get to the bathroom by yourself when you're completely stoned on narcotics.

If you do any of the above, your PA has 5,123 patients, and since you're being a dumbass, whatever stupid thing you did will go to your doctors. Check out of the hospital ASAP…you're done for.

Name tags / embroidered emblems

Checking emblems or name tags is fun, but totally unnecessary. You'll only remember one, or perhaps two, of the staff who walk in and out of your room per day because—again—you're on drugs. Trust me, there're a million staff members with name tags. Ok, it's comforting and all to know each staff member has a title and you wouldn't want it to read, "Some Guy," but…let it go.

Added point:

Hospitals put name badges in the wrong place. You want to read who they are so you can say, "Good morning, Mary," but they put the name tag on their left or right breast. No matter what your gender, it's awkward. Your motives are entirely honorable, but when you even slightly attempt to see their name and rubberneck a look at their badge, you're immediately an oversexed, inappropriate, nasty old fart. It's difficult. Why don't you put it on their crotch or ass ?!@! Jeeeessss! Put the damn name tag on their side pocket or something! Yes, you cannnn try the "Good morning, ma'am" or "Good morning, sir" approach, but that gets even worse when you pick the wrong gender. This happened to me. Nurse walked in my room to do something and I let out a friendly, "Well hello, sir!" Nurse came back with a husky, "Name's Darlene." Just let whomever do whatever to your whatchamacallit—you'll be ok.

Code Whatever

Evidently hospital staff must keep a code recognition list in their waistband underneath those nifty blue gowns/scrubs/rubs. A code list explanation of all the hospital codes covering each and every damn thing that could ever go wrong in a hospital. There's a code color for when they're serving mystery meat meatloaf in the cafeteria, a code color for flatulence, and a code color—yellow or brown—depending on the bowel issue. You know these code deals, you've seen hospital/doctor TV shows. !@#$#@!" (alarm going off)—STAFF ALERT! STAFF ALERT! We have a code beige in Room 749 (staff running around with a WTF look)! I repeat, code beige in Room 749! (staff checking their code list, but can't find it!@#!) What the hell is code beige?! Shit! "All staff respond! All staff respond!!"

Whilst in the hospital, you will hear tons of these code-color alerts. Stay away from a code brown. Trust me on this; no details.

The Stethoscope Maneuver

This phenomenon is closely related to the Poke Your Stomach Maneuver, which I'll get to in a minute. The Stethoscope Maneuver occurs every time a doctor or PA comes in your room. It goes like this: Knock on the door (to make sure your pants aren't down), doctor or PA walks in and says, "Hi. I'm Dr. Beatlecowshiwitz from EchoCardioland, and, if you would, please remove your warm/cozy/ shirt/blouse and let me send you through the roof by putting this ice-cold metal circle on your skin."

First off, do they keep those in a freezer? What's the deal with every doctor in the whole universe having to listen to your back and chest with a stethoscope—every single time? If you have the gout and your big toe is the size of an artichoke, they'll come in and listen to your chest. If you say the walls are talking to you, they listen to your chest. I swear, if a doctor walks by you on the street, they'll say, "Excuse me," and listen to your chest!

Some patients in our lung transplant forum have come up with a "stetho-conspiracy theory." Hospitals have doctors perform the Stetho Maneuver so said hospital can say you were examined. Think about it, if they walked in, looked at you, and said, "Yep, well, you look ok," and left, how could the hospital bill you? "Ah, excuse me, billing department, but the doctor didn't...like...do anything. He came in and just said, 'Hi.'"

Billing department, "Yes, we get that, but she did examine you with a stethoscope, and those aren't cheap."

Our forum group is onto something. It would be different if the Stetho Maneuver only happened once in a while. One time this group of doctors with interns came into my room. Tromp, tromp, tromp. One immediately started the famous Stetho Maneuver. Ok, fine. Butttt then, the remaining three did the sameeee damn thing!! One right after another!! I wanted to yell, "Hey, huddle up and confer with each other. Ask each other, what did you hear?" "I didn't hear nothin'." "I think he farted." Thennn, you get four bills! "But, they all listened, sir." Conspiracy.

The Poke Your Stomach Maneuver

Very similar to the Stetho Maneuver, a doctor and PA walk in your room introducing themselves and ask you to remove your shirt. Hopefully your shirt, not your blue gown which exposes everything. Then they say, "Please, if you would, lie down on this lounge." The "lounge"—which is certainly a stretch of the imagination— has a cold, crispy, cream-colored sort of parchment paper covering an old, dilapidated, cracked, pseudo leather examination bench/ table. It evidently bends in three places and has uncomfortable creases in all the wrong spots. This plank is also slightly on an angle so the whole time you're up on it, you're slowly sliding downhill. This is when the Poke Your Stomach maneuver begins. The doctor slowly starts poking your stomach in a weird way while looking at the ceiling. "Does thissss hurt?" Why do they look up at the ceiling? What does the ceiling have to do with it? Moving to a different spot on your stomach, no matter what your answer was to the first question, they ask, "Any discomfort over here?" More viewing the ceiling. You answer, "Nope…actually I'm here for my toe."

The doctor says, "Well, yes, your toe, I know. We always need to do a little poking around though, don't we!" Same conspiracy.

Calling the financial department, I ask, "What am I being billed for?"

The secretary says, "Stomach poking."

I say, "Oh, so I'm being billed $1,234 for stomach poking for my toe problem. Not sure why I even asked."

Secretary says in a cheery voice, "Thankkkk youuuu." and hangs up.

ICU

Ok, here's the way serious place. This area is like Greek mythology—the River Styx. People with masks, knives, clampers, picks, saws, the whole nine yards. This is the mysterious, scary, dim, cold, and spooky place. Do not, whatever you do, crack a joke in the ICU. Don't ask for anything, no water, no bedpan. ICU doesn't believe in bowel movements—they're too busy. Remember they said don't eat anything for forty days before your surgery? Same people. Don't even move. Stare straight ahead. No questions, comments, or sounds. If they ask, "When were you born?" don't say anything. You're probably completely out anyway. This is the intense place. It's even in the title: "Intensive" care unit. ICU also stands for: "I Can Unfix you…if I want…don't fuck with me; I'm not kidding."

Another name for ICU is "I—See—U." It's kind of like the Robert DeNiro thing again. This time it's two fingers pointing at your eyes and then back at his. Stay still like a rabbit. Don't even move your eyes around.

You think I'm making this up. I'm not. Even the machines look scary. You know the movie, *Lucy*, where they remake Scarlett Johansson into a killer robot or some damn thing? Ol' Scarlett is hooked up to all these machines going in and out of her body to make her bionic. ICU is just like that. I'm not kidding. Robot claws menacing towards you, TV screens blipping, wires going nowhere to make it look cool, tubes going everywhere—I hate tubes. Tubes always have to do with weird shit. Say "tube" out loud by itself. Sounds weird. And they strap you down in all sorts of configurations. One time they taped my head so far sideways on the table I was like, "Heyyy! Yo!! My neck is like cramping really, really bad here, and you think I'm out, but I'm not because I just heard you're meeting each other at the bar after this!@#!"

I'd never want to work in an ICU. They all walk around with little, pursed smiles because they're being intense. They walk with their legs tight together because they're afraid to pass gas.

When you have nothing to do in your wheelchair or you're being trucked around the hospital on a gurney, observe other areas. The staff smiles. They actually laugh, tell stories, and joke, even walk around with a Starbucks coffee. In the ICU, if someone even chuckles, the whole ward turns and glares at them. Heaven forbid if a nurse drops a scalpel—clang!! Everyone in the whole ICU would shit at the same time.

Very, very uptight place. You're saying, "It damn well should be!" but wow!! It makes a library look like an amusement park. I mean, I was there and it's a damn good thing someone didn't say, "Hey, what's that thing hanging out of your dick?" I would have laughed really hard out loud and had my stomach tubes come spraying out like a Mr. Slinky garden nozzle.

Nurses/Staff Point of View

I feel quite obligated to add this staff side of things, a.k.a. staff perspective, because, certainly, there's another side. There always is.

The hospital staff members work hard. Their job is not an ordinary one like delivering Fritos to a party store. It's difficult stuff. I dare anyone to tell me nurses and staff don't earn their pay. The entire staff: the gurney drivers dealing with patients in pain; nurses trying to get someone from their bed to a gurney without making them pass out; the desk workers trying to keep all the hospital lingo/jangle/appointments straight with sick, ornery patients and pressured doctors hovering over them; the cleaning crew—OMG.

Nurses knock on the door aaaas they walk in your room. Thangs ta do! Got ten more of the same next hour! First of all, they've seen it—butt, dick, sagging whatever—every crack from here to the Grand Canyon. Hey, they're nurses. They make the whole place work.

My hat is off to all of them. Ok, more than my hat, but that's a strange image. I always tried to thank the staff for whatever job they were executing around me. Executing—probably not a good word choice—but whether it was poking me with a needle or prod, making me do weird exercises, getting me to eat hospital food, bed-washing me with a sponge like I do my car, or taking an arduous journey to the bathroom with me, they did it.

BP

You're thinking "blood pressure," right? These acronyms aren't always what you think. Nurse strolls in and says, "How y'all doin? I'm taking your BP." You stick out your arm so she can wrap the plastic sleeve around and take your blood pressure. She says, "Noooo, your bedpan! You don' fill it the whole way, darlin'." Don't trust acronyms.

MRIs

Big, white, tube-like machine they slide you in and then go to lunch. If you're claustrophobic, forgit 'bout itttt! If you do actually make it all the way in the tube before freaking out, it will start to tick really loud and the attendant/mechanic running the MRI—who is behind bulletproof glass, BTW—will tell you to ignore it. He'll say, kind of in this faraway echo-type voice, "Ticking's just a gigantic magnet sucking things out of your body. No metal plates in your head or shrapnel floating around, right? You might explode, so just letting you know."

Bulletproof glass is disconcerting. Why should I be in an area where other human beans are behind bulletproof glass? It's the same with x-rays. You stand in front of this metal plate naked, but the attendant is covered with lead like he's in *Game of Thrones*. Doesn't anyone question stuff like this? If someone came in a room and put an octopus on your head and stood back holding a spear gun, would you ask why?

Heart ECHO

"ECHO" stands for something, but just know this is the jelly room. They smear KY Jelly all over your chest. Nurse will then take this cold—similar to the doctor's stethoscope—wand and start running it all around your body whilst looking at some kind of bluish screen that's humming. She or he will make sounds like, "Um hmmm, aaaah, um hmmm." This is actually one of the more fun tests because you see your heart beat on this old TV set monitor.

Pretty odd experience. You're lying sideways on this table and your cheek is all mushed in on a pillow (the cheek next to your nose, that is). You're talking out of the side of your mouth like the Joker to this stranger gazing at your heart. Dub, dub...dub, dub. Your very own heart! So, this person, who looks extremely bored, is nonchalantly looking at what's keeping you alive, right? Very Frankensteinish. The silence becomes too much and you finally say, "Ah, how's the ol' heart beating there...ahhh..." straining to see his nurse badge, "Ed?"

All these ECHO techs use this "circle and hold" deal with their wand. The metal wand in their hand...never mind. Circle...and hold. Circle and hold. Then they stop and there's all sorts of clicking noises. Ed does the circle and hold again and stares intently at the screen. He doesn't respond to your question. Maybe Ed doesn't want to talk. He smears more KY. Surprisingly, after what seems like twenty minutes, Ed says, "Excuse me?"

To be fair, Ed has a very specific and intricate job. It's not like he's flipping pancakes, so I said, "Sorry, I shouldn't interrupt while you're looking at my very own heart there…Just sort of wondering what you're seeing?"

Again, Ed doesn't say anything. I start getting worried. Maybe there's a ping-pong ball in there, maybe my heart has no valves. But Ed finally says, after another ten minutes, "There's a blank area around here." My neck is cramping so I can't see.

"But your linear vortex inside the ventricular heart valve is byopit-cranialogically chronosated to the outer wall in its relationship to inner sanctum five revolving around the MPH factor on your credit card."

Ok, he didn't say that, but it's what it sounded like. So, then I asked, "Um…is that blank area a bad thing?"

"Oh, no," he offers, "that's just the jelly." Click.

You can ask more, but there's a damn good chance you won't understand the answer. They do this on purpose. It's brilliant. It gets you to stop asking questions. Remember, you're the eighty-fifth person to pose the same "How am I doin' there?" question. I mean he couldddd say, "Your valve is acting funny," but no, it's got to have all the messed-up medical lingo / code / weird stuff to make you stop. The lingo is impressive, even if they're just making it up. Besides, Ed can't make any medical interpretations anyway, because he's not the doctor. So, there's that.

Buzz, click, zap. "Yep, got it," Ed says as he stands up. "The doctor will go over the test results with you. Use this towel to clean up that jelly on your chest."

When's the last time someone said that…. hmmm? Don't answer.

EWT: Esophagus Wire Test

Now, this test did not go well. It wasn't good for me, and not good for others.

Some people may deal with this test just fine, but I didn't. My lung transplant team head nurse, Kristen, who took on the challenge of taking care of me for life, told me what they were going to do with this fun test.

After reading this you might question its validity, but, please, for the sake and sanity of all involved, the following is all true.

My EWT test involves running a "thin" wire up my nose, down the back of my throat, past my esophagus, and into my stomach. Hmmm. She mentioned it wouldn't take long and the testers/ testes/testo people would numb my throat so I wouldn't feel a thing.

Ok, important juncture: Understand what doctors, nurses, aides, and gurney drivers tell you isn't always true. In hospitals, secretaries tell the truth. Everyone else fogs up the story. Yes, fibs float around hospitals like Cheerios in too much milk. It's not the staff's fault—they have to slant material; they're instructed to. Ever hear the saying, "The truth could kill you"? Well…it could. Think about it. They can't say, "Yeah, you're going down to this weird-ass room, someone in a Freddy Krueger mask is going to stick a long copper wire down your throat and tape the end of it to your nose like a dangling fishing lure so people can laugh at you. Oh, and just so you know, the eight-foot wire will be in your stomach hanging around for a couple of days making you sick."

Answer: I—don't—think so!! Whomever would say ok to that would be one pistachio short of a nuthouse.

Thus, as nineteenth century poet Emily Dickenson put it, the staff was slanting the truth. This quaint verbal exercise is quite common these days in our political circles, so you're probably used to it.

Calling these instructions/explanations "lies" isn't fair, though. There are always times when you slant the truth. When your partner walks out of a store dressing room in a new outfit and asks, "Does this make me look fat?" you slant the truth. When someone spends hours in the kitchen making their special recipe involving beets, even though you don't like beets, you say they taste great. Got to, sometimes.

What happened to me with this EWT test covers slanting, switching, vice, graft, greasing ball bearings, and one really, really pissed-off female gastroenterologist doctor we'll call Dr. Gastro.

Gastroenterologist sounds really bad. It starts with "gastro," which is very similar to "ghastly," moves to "enter" which means "go into" something, and finishes with the famous "gist." It wasn't going to be good from the git-go.

During my in-hospital testing stay, Dr. Gastro winged into my room. She was nice looking, short, and had sort of a sharp angled nose pointing downward. Her blond hair was cut off sharply at the shoulder and she had black-rimmed glasses. The ice cube stethoscope hit my chest and I jumped, as usual. She listened, looking at the ceiling. No "hello," no "how are ya," no "nice chest," nothing. After doing the proverbial listening, Dr. Gastro leaned back and robotically said, "You'll go to eighth floor for EWT."

Dr. Gastro reminded me of my nasty math teacher in elementary school who failed me five straight years. I sensed it. She entered the room the same exact way. My math teacher hated me—probably for good reason—but Dr. Gastro had just met me!

"Ishmael takes you to procedure." She eliminated words like "the" to save time evidently. "After procedure, make sure you're not active this evening (like I was going to go play hockey), and we take probe out same time tomorrow, measuring acid reflux twenty-four-hour period." Maybe she's Russian. Then she said, "View you tomorrow," like I was a museum exhibit. Out she went for her robust Starbucks and out I went to the wire-rooters.

Once at the procedure area, you wait in this room with white curtains for about twenty minutes. Sometime there's groaning going on on the other side, which could be a lot of things. Finally, a nurse sashays in and says what they all say, "We're going to numb (pick an area) so it will make the procedure easier for you." Two things come to mind with this little quip. One: When the numbness wears off, then what? Two: Sometimes numbing said area is worse than the procedure. Case in point: penis, scrotum, etc. Three: If my throat is all numb drunk, how am I going to swallow? Minor issue.

The male nurse also adds, "When I do this, it will taste like sulphur, like rotten eggs."

Wait. We can go to the moon, walk around a space capsule one hundred thousand gazillion miles away waving to the camera, but no one can figure out how to make some liquid shit taste like peppermint?

Suddenly, a hoard of staff with masks arrive. They stretch this large rubber condom across my mouth, holding my lips open like I'm the guy in the *Scream* painting. Then, they start sticking this— no kidding—copper wire up my nose and down my now semi-useless, numbed-up throat. Bim, bam, done, and they all walk away. Fini, zip, and zap. I thought to myself, *That must have been one pretty short wire. Cool.* This line of thinking would come back to haunt me later.

What happened next takes place around five p.m. on Fridays in every hospital around the country. Everyone leaves—staff, bean counters, visitors, semi-visitors, and mice. Ok, not everyone, but almost. Work stations are vast wastelands.

Rule 34: If you're going to get sick, don't get sick on a weekend. What little staff left working the weekend are on hold mode until Monday. They won't tell you that, but they are.

Jackie and Zachera decided they had to drive back to our house in Boyne City that particular Friday, because driving down we had no idea we would be staying in Chicago, let alone a hospital, for any length of time. Things happened so fast. You kind of need a lot of clothes, underwear, and stuff when staying anywhere for more than two days, so off they headed on a six-hour drive. It was six hours "in good weather," as we say in the north, and it was snowing to beat the band, which didn't bode well. Nevertheless, even though it was a semi-bad idea, they felt they had to go.

The lung transplant team was getting closer to a judgment on whether or not I could be placed on the national organ donor list. The problem was the decision couldn't be made right away because there were still more tests to be completed. Conversely, because my health was going downhill fast, they didn't think they could wait any longer. Because of all this consternation, the transplant team wanted me in close proximity at all times. Their decision, one way or another, would affect where Jackie and I stayed because the team needed me within fifteen minutes of MMHMMM. In a big city, that means quite close because of traffic, Ubers, subways, taxis, pastrami sandwiches, etc. We might be in Chicago for an indefinite length of time. "Indefinite" is a disturbing word.

Zachera and Jackie felt they could drive all the way back to Boyne City, pack up as much as possible, attend Grandpa's birthday, and head back in our GMC Terrain. Even though the weather didn't look good in terms of snow and wind, they headed out because, as Jackie said, "We just can't stay here with nothing at all! We need clothes, everything, you name it! We didn't count on this—who knew? We'll have to 'go on, come back.'" This was a phrase we always used ever since a Jamaican cab driver said it to us. "You won' ride, mon? We go on, come back. Irie."

Jackie's eyes told more than she was saying as they slowly left my room, waving goodbye. She knew the gravity of the situation. This was not going well. After they were gone, I thought no matter what happens, this is going to be difficult for them. It already was. I so didn't want this, but it was now out of my control.

Gazing out from my room overlooking the tall downtown Chicago buildings and giant Lake Michigan, I felt extremely down. I was worried because I knew what a dangerous drive Zachera and Jackie were taking. We had been there; driving on an expressway in the middle of a complete snow whiteout is unnerving. Accidents would be all around them. This was all my fault. I could stop the whole thing and just give it up. Maybe I'd live longer than they thought. You hear about it. But this wasn't that kind of sick. I was in a negative spiral.

As it started to get darker outside, the city lights started to show like evening stars. Sitting in this sort of old brown bay window with a wire dangling from my nose, three things ran around in my mind. One: *This wire sucks and is extremely uncomfortable.* Two: *Should I, could I, go through with all this?* Three: This was going to be a two-day fun fest—floated facetiously. It wasn't going to be fun at all. *No one's around, terrible food, and can't swallow worth shit due to the EWT wire. What a party weekend.*

Sitting in a lump with such happy thoughts, I was silent for quite a while. The city lights were now in full bloom and the view was actually beautiful. The city never ceased to amaze me. How could they build all that? Who figures that all out? Why didn't it all sink into the ground on top of the subway cars? What if you're on the top floor and something terrible happens? Fun, fun mood.

There were some flashing lights directly below my seventh-floor window on the street. I hadn't really noticed them before. Red and green lights were emanating from a marquee spelling out Gino's East. Considering how bad I was feeling, the Gino's East sign was like a mirage.

I'm alone, everyone's gone, there's nothing to do, my hospital dinner is going to be an attempt at best. Bummer of a depressed state.

Looking down on the street below, cars created meandering snakes of light. I noticed the Gino's sign again. Huh. A beer would chum things up a bit, I supposed. More importantly, a Chicago-style pizza pairs well with beer. If you know Chicago, you know Gino's. You also know Chicago pizzas are almost three inches thick and The Meat Lovers will have about a one-inch layer of pepperoni!

Fine, if you want to be a vegetarian, I totally honor your thoughts. Go green, go veggies. But I'm a carnivore and always will be. In cavepeople times, I would be the Clan member wearing deerskin and tie-up foot pads, sitting next to the fire eating a five-pound leg of yak.

These new thoughts were making me feel slightly better—food always did. The prospect of getting a Gino's Meat Lovers deep-dish pizza from the marquee restaurant and somehow into my room sounded really good, but unattainable. But I truly had nothing to do, and, in a strange way, my idea seemed like a challenge. Getting a beer along with it was also outlandish, but was worth a try.

Hitting the old call button on the creamy yellow remote with cracks in it, I tried to find out if anyone was left on the seventh floor. Maybe I could get the last person living on Earth to answer.

After a couple of minutes, a warped voice answered the yucky walkie-talkie thing, "Kcccsssss…crackle…kccsssss…Hello, yesssss, ksseessscicccc...." You would think I was David Bowie's Major Tom calling in for the last time from outer space. I quickly said, "Ah, yes...um...this is room 782. Robert Emmet – April 6th, 1950." They ask your birthdate no matter who is doing what. Once, when I said "Hello" to a familiar employee in the hospital's first floor coffee shop, he turned and said, "Date of birth?" I mean, it's bad. When you approach a hospital urinal, a robotic voice says, "Enter—birth-date—move closer—go."

Evidently the only nurse in all of Chicago finally answered the phone. "Seven-eight-two—I knowwww y'all's room number, honey, I's talkin' to it."

The nurse's response was a bit snarky, but I nicely said, "Ha, well, I guess you do...are you...well...um...would...or...could you send someone down for a sec?"

"Wat you need?"

No way I was going to tell the front desk!! So, I said, "I'll have to explain when they get here. It's kind of...you know...embarrass-ing." That would get her! Nurses secretly love gnarly stuff. They told me they did. One said, "Why else would we go into nursing?"

"Click" was the only sound that came back. They don't spend much time talking on those speaker/wand deals. Sometimes the speaker/wand would answer back, "Parking lot five, what's the problem?" It was the parking lot attendant from across the street. Must have been some kind of a technical issue. Weird stuff like that happens in the hospitals.

Quite a few minutes later, emphasis on "quite," a young, tall nurse knocked on my door and walked in. "I'm Jennie. I'll be your night nurse." She was somewhat athletic looking, about twenty-six years old, maybe, with light brown hair pulled back in the prover-bial nurse's ponytail. She had strong arms like she worked out. Not weightlifting strong, more like swimmer or pole-vaulter strong.

I said, "So you're one of the chosen few here tonight? Just you, that's it? You and a couple others somewhere have to take care of the whole floor?"

"Nope. Allie will be helping me. She's new...in training. I have to show her the ropes." And at that, Allie walked in. "This is Allie. Allie, Mr. Emmet." Allie was taller than Jennie, thin, had large black glasses, fashionable lately, sort of hipster. She had jet black curly hair. It stuck out quite a bit, like she tried for a style and it didn't cooperate.

I said, "So, this is going to be one big happy party on the ol' seventh floor, eh?" laughing. Little did I know.

Looking at Allie, Jennie said with a wry smile, "Yep. Nothing but fun up here alll night long!" Allie rolled her eyes in sarcastic agreement. Jennie asked, "What can we help you with?"

How to get these two nurses to be complicit with me and my nose-to-throat-to-stomach-wire pizza idea? I said, "Well, as you can see, I've got this copper wire deal in my nose and down somewhere and I'm very uncomfortable and…um…that tray with tonight's hospital dinner…is…well…more than unattractive."

Neither of them said anything. They kept looking at me as if I was going to say more. Finally, Jennie said, "Yessss," holding it out. Of course, they knew exactly where I was going.

I went on, "You see, I hate bothering you, but .. .ah…this has been a rough day…hospital food…and I was hoping someone could step up to the plate here." I wasn't getting any response. Nothing. Allie started cleaning up a side table with plastic breathing appliances on it. Jennie was still looking at me, waiting.

Drastic times called for drastic measures. Squinting my eyes, I said slowly, "Do you think…ah" I paused, then said fast, "If no one knew, could you two smuggle a Gino's pizza up to my room? It's right below us down on the street there. I could give you the money and we could share it. You've got to be hungry, right? I'll even pay you for your trouble."

Jennie and Allie looked at each other. Jennie smirked, "Wellll, I don't know, Allie. It might take a lot of money to persuade us to take a chanceeee like thatttt. Bring a pizza allll the way up here past the guards, the main desk?"

Allie laughed, "Breaking every rule in the book."

I quickly said, "Noooo. They wouldn't fire…"

Jennie interrupted laughing, "Just kidding, Mr. Emmet, it's not against any rules. We do it all the time. What kind of pizza would you like?"

I couldn't believe it! I thought it was a long shot, at best.

"Really?!"

They both nodded.

"Cool!" and doing my best Jim Carrey impression, "Alrighty thennnn!! Ah...I suppose getting a six pack of beer is..."

"Don't push it...but we can get you some Pepsi or something." Allie grabbed some paper off the desk and acted like a server, "Your order pleaseeee?" They were fun and trying to make the best out of a long night.

"You guys get what you want on it. All I need is lots of pepperoni!" I said, as forgotten tape held forgotten wire leading to a forgotten place. All was overshadowed by Gino's. I was throwing hell to the wind.

Jennie said, "I love pepperoni."

"No kidding! Get the Meat Lover's Special!" I said, feeling much better than earlier.

Jennie answered, "Fine by me. How about you, Allie?"

Allie looked like a vegetarian to me, so I thought piles of pepperoni might throw her, but she didn't even blink. "Sounds great."

"Here's some money. If it's not enough, come back and I'll give you whatever."

Now, keep in mind, the purpose of the fun EWT wire in my nose was for testing acid reflux and to find out if my esophagus was ok. If the test indicated a problem—like too much acid—they would have to put final testing on hold and fix it. Being put on hold meant not being put on the national donor list, pure and simple. The tape fastened to the test wire and stuck firmly on front of my nose prevented said wire from sliding back down my throat. All in all, a fashionable look. Just want to give you the complete image and situation here. And, no, I was not thinking straight.

Over an hour later (come on, it's the city), Jennie knocked and yelled, "Gino's, at your service!" The seventh floor must have been really devoid of staff and patients, because Jennie wouldn't have said it so loudly otherwise. Allie walked in behind her with a cold two-liter of Pepsi, and cups. Jennie sat the square box with a steaming Chicago-style Gino's pizza down on the table next to the bay window. Fun, as opposed to my un-fun week.

Allie and Jennie said, almost together, "We've got work to do. You enjoy your dinner and we'll stop by later to have some with you, ok?"

"I will, to say the least! But a bunch of this is for you guys, ya know."

"Have what you want. If there're leftovers." Jennie winked. "we'll be gladddd to get rid of them for you." They turned and went out, shutting the door.

There I sat, eating pizza and drinking Pepsi, which didn't seem to bother my stomach at all. Surprisingly, I could swallow pretty well. I was making chicken salad out of chickenshit. The reason for the EWT test had conveniently escaped my mind—conveniently—whilst romping through crunchy crust, oozing blends of cheese, and heaps of pepperoni, as advertised. We, as human beans, function in twenty-four-hour cycles. Looking further out than what's in front of us at the moment doesn't always happen.

After the nurses came by and finished the last few pieces of pizza, we talked about their jobs and training, the Chicago Cubs, and their favorite restaurants—always a great topic in Chicago. Jennie told Allie they had to get back to work, so we both thanked each other, and they headed out to spend their evening changing bandages and making patients who could walk the halls. I was more than full.

About an hour later, whilst watching some soccer game, I noticed something acid-like come up in my throat. No big deal. I took a drink of watered-down lemonade sitting on the white swivel stand and went on watching. A few minutes later, I noticed the same sensation. This time it was more pronounced. Soccer announcers with English accents were fun to listen to compared to our football-announcer talking heads.

"Heee cranked heeees shot a bit lift. Sidewinder, I'll tell you. He's macking a statement, he is." The other announcer agreed, "Landcaster's a good'n true. Chriminage sod him a bill a goods an eee tok the bait…Eee took the bait."

I could listen to those broadcasters all night. However, acid in my stomach wasn't taking all night; it was right now. Pepperoni heartburn. I knew it, heartburn…but didn't expect it to hit me so hard. Gee…a wire in my stomach. It occurred to me far too late the wire in my stomach was now going to send me off the charts for acid reflux.

As my heartburn amped up, I started to panic. *This test has to go. They'll never understand. I told them I never get heartburn, which was true. I could eat all sorts of spicy dishes, and nothing. It must have been the wire causing it. Ok, the pepperoni didn't help, but I could eat a whole pepperoni pizza and never get an upset stomach, let alone acid problems.* They were going to read my test and get a false result!@#!"

Took two Rolaids at nine p.m., to no avail. By ten p.m., it was really bad. My mind was whirring, *I have to do something. If the wire isn't in my stomach and throat, no acid levels, no esophagus problems. It's got to come out. It's the only way. They'll never know. I'll just lay it by my bed, covered up so the night nurses won't see it. I'll be sleeping; they won't check my nose. Then, in the morning, I'll say the wire got really uncomfortable and worked its way out on its own. The wire was short, as far as I could tell. One yank and it would come out. It might hurt but it was worth it. I've gone through so many tests and procedures and passed them all. I can't let this one EWT thing blow make my chances.*

It seemed pretty quiet in the hallways, around one a.m., and Jennie and Allie had already checked on me. I listened. Sometimes you could hear the nurses or aides talking or moving apparatus, but it was silent. I got a towel from the bathroom in case my brilliant idea went south, sat down on the chair by the window, and planned my move.

I'll take the adhesive tape off my nose, get a good grip on the wire, take as big a breath as I can muster, and quickly jerk the short amount of wire out. Simple.

Ok, here we go. The adhesive tape on my nose was stuck firmly to the end of the wire. They had left a small amount of excess wire in a loop outside my nose, presumably for doing exactly what I was about to do. Winding the extra wire around the index finger of my right hand, I calmed myself as much as I could, took a big breath, and yanked. The wire started coming out! It's going to work! But the wire kept coming. *How ——ing long is this thing! Shitttt!!* I kept pulling and pulling—whattt the hellll!! Finally, the wire's end came flying out of my nose, spraying my face, and dangling all over the place! Aaarrrrr ... Goddamn thing was three feet long! They told me it was "short, just down your throat." I was thinking nine, ten inches! ——ing thing was long! @#! Could have wired my kitchen with it!@#. I shivered, thinking, *Thatttt could have been wayyyy bad.*

After taking stock, I seemed alright, didn't feel too bad. My throat and nose were sore, but I was ok. Actually, I was thankful I didn't kill myself. It worked, though—no emergencies—no blood—no nurses. With my heart pounding, I put my oxygen canola back on and thought, *So, alright...whoa...that was close. Dealing with the nurses won't be that bad though; I mean, they might not even know.*

The wire! My first thought was, *if they see it's gone or lying on the bed, they'll say, "What the hell !???!@#"* So, I wound the wire up as tight as I could and slipped it into the middle pages of a two-year-old *National Geographic* magazine—a fitting place. I went back to sleep.

Around 6:30 a.m. or so, Jennie and Allie knocked on the door to check on me before their shift ended. Of course, they woke me up, like they do.

What's with that?! You're sick, feel terrible, hot, shitty, cold, bleary eyed, saggy...and you justttt fell asleep and...what do you know... Bam!! Nurses turn on all the lights and you jump up from fright. This, I found out, happens every three hours throughout the night.

They come in and ask you how you're feeling. *Well, now that I'm awake…let's see…um…not good…crappy…yep…that would sum it up. Gettin' some sleep would have helped, but I know, it's policy, but isn't the point of trying to get better, trying to get better?*

Jennie said, "Good morning, Robert, we need to take your blood pressure and temperature."

"Ok," I said, in a fog. Allie went through the motions. No mention of my now wireless nose. Allie's BP packet tightened on my upper arm, and Jennie said, "Have you had a bowel movement?" Allie watched the dial for the BP.

Now, there you go. This is the kind of thing that makes the whole hospital experience so damn weird and fun. Think about it. I had a fairly normal life, blew leaves, cut the lawn, spent time with friends, watched movies, the usual. Now, it's the middle of the night in some mammoth downtown building, I'm hiding an esophagus wire in a magazine, have on a nightgown that lets all of Chicago see the lumber yard, and have two young, really nice-looking women asking me about my bowel movements.

As I started to answer, Allie said, "Jennie, where's his EWT wire?" Shit…

Of course they were going to notice; it's just if my mind thought it was a good thing to do in the first place, certainly it made sense to visualize everyone completely missing a wire hanging from my nose. Making a face like a guy who's just had a cop ask, "Whose cocaine is that lying on the car seat?" Kind of a shrug, kind of disbelief, kind of "I'm so ——ing screwed."

Jennie immediately said, "Where's your nose wire?" Simple, direct, getting right to the damn point, the "you're in trouble" approach.

Saying "I don't know" seemed lame. Since I had broken pizza with them the night before, it might work but probably wouldn't be nice to push things. The doctor maybe—but not them. Besides, they were young and smart. Also, there was a slight chance they might get in trouble with the brass, seeing as it happened on their watch. My mind slipped to *That's it, it's their fault!* but I couldn't throw them under the bus (which is a pretty gross saying when you think about it). I could pull a damn wire out of my ass, but couldn't do that. I quickly said, "The damn thing hurt and I was getting sick from it and I couldn't sleep and there weren't any good movies on and Oswald didn't shoot Kennedy."

"Where did you put it?" Allie asked.

"It's in the *National Geographic* magazine there on the table." This was taking me back to my grade school days of getting in trouble. Their attitude was similar to the nuns, but in this case, they were nice and weren't going to hit me.

"Why is your nose wire in a magazine?" Jennie peered at me.

I absolutely hate negative rhetorical questions. There's always someone asking those kind of questions—questions they already know the damn answer to. Trick questions. If you don't come up with the right answer—which was no answer at all—you were in trouble.

I said to the nurses, "That 'nose wire / magazine' question is.... Well...how much time do you have?"

Jennie wasn't laughing, and either was Allie. In a louder voice, Jennie said, "Dr. Fastenyourseatbelts is going to be soooo furious at you!"

Allie looked at Jennie and said, "Are we going to get in trouble for this?"

Jennie came back with, "No, but he is."

"Why on earth did you do that?" Allie asked.

"I don't know...it's just...that pizza...awful heart burn...acid reflux numbers sky high .. .and doctor what's-her-face and her graphs. She'll report them to Dr. Anisee and then no lung donor list."

Jennie replied, completely ignoring my pseudo justification, "How the hell did you get the wire out?"

"I thought it was really short."

"You could have really hurt yourself," Allie said.

"I know, damn wire was wayyyy longer than I thought. But, put yourself in my undies, would you chance being taken off a transplant donor list because of pepperoni pizza?"

Allie said to Jennie, "He's got a point."

Jennie said, "Point or no point, they're going to be angry! And... they're going to make you do that test all over again today."

"Well, I don't have heartburn now, so I'll put up with it. I took about a bottle of Rolaids."

"I'll page the doctor; she's on call," Allie said, and left the room. I looked at Jennie and said, "I had no choice."

"You had a lot of choices...Jesus...I'd like to be empathetic, but you can't do stuff like that. Why didn't you call us like we told you?"

"Because you wouldn't have done it. You wouldn't be allowed to. I was the only one who could do it."

"Well, speaking of screwed, the doctor is on her way." Jennie and Allie quickly left and said, "Good luck" in an ominous tone. I didn't blame them for getting as far away from my room as they could. If Doctor FrankenFurious called the main desk for Jennie and Allie's explanation, they wanted the speaker in my room to squawk, "ah...I'm...(hiss)...somewhere with...(blip)...patients."

Within minutes, in walked Gastro doc. She didn't even get to the side of my bed. "The front desk said you pulled out your EWT? Whatttt were you thinking?" (There it was...I knew it!) "I've never had anyone ever do that in fifteen years. Why in the world did you do that?"

This time it wasn't rhetorical; she really wanted to know. Med hallucinations might have worked. But I actually started to tell her the truth and...bam!

"When did you do this?"

"Somewhere in the middle of the night, maybe one a.m. It's not the nurses' fault. Entirely my doing. When they saw the wire was gone, they immediately called you." No bus from me.

Dr. Smiley grabbed her clipboard, scribbled something, made a beeline towards the door, then stopped and said, "You will be scheduled in an hour for the same test. It will be another twenty-four hours, you know. This time, leave wire in!"

Doing my impression of Arnold Schwarzenegger saying, "I'llll be bokkk" didn't seem like a good idea.

In about twenty minutes, Jennie and Allie snuck back in after checking to see if anyone was lurking in the hall.

"Are you two on tonight's work schedule?" I asked.

Jennie replied, "Nope. Rest time! It was fun meeting you. Well... interesting. Remember, do what they say. No tricks, ok?" They both waved as they left.

The staff did come get me for another EWT test. They rolled me into the same procedure department for the repeat performance. The nurse, per usual, said, "Robert Emmet, April 6th, 1950?" again.

I said, "Yes, correct."

Then the male nurse, who was looking closely at my chart, peered at me and said, "Ohhhh, hey, wait! You're that guy! The guy who pulled out his EWT wire all by himself last night! Crazy! Everyone in the hospital is talking about you—great story!! What made you do it?!"

Great...infamous...So pleased to make the hospital's Hall of Fame! @#! I didn't say anything. The nurse laughed and said, "I've never heard of anyone having the...ah...guts to do that. Wow. Pulled it right out, eh? You must be pretty tough."

On one of those tiny slits of white paper, my fortune cookie read:

"If you want the rainbow, you have to tolerate the rain."

14

Nurses, Questions, and Dirty Jobs

Nurses and their jobs—cops and doughnuts. Consider your job and what you actually physically and mentally do day after day. Then, think about being a nurse and having patients ask you the same damn questions all day long, along with other fun stuff like finding out when you had a bowel movement.

Don't you just love that question: "Ahhhh...um...let's see, I always discuss my bowel movements with anyone who shows up. Actually, I was just talking to a bank teller down on Michigan Ave. about my last undertaking. She thought it was good I was regular. I mean, things were going pretty well in the fart department at seven a.m....so I took a crap at eight a.m....it was pretty impressive, but whoa...after they gave me milk of magnesia at ten a.m.... all hell broke loose." (Milk of magnesia: what a gross name. What is it? What or who got milked?)

They really are going to ask you, "When was your last bowel movement?" Come onnnn! Isn't anything sacred? Hospitals/doctors can't make everything perfect for you. Certainly not all the time. Like many things in life, it's a rollercoaster ride. So, you have to be prepared for the dips, milks, and movements.

Alright, bathroom issues. There are only a few other things you do in this world as private as "Whaaaa we're talkin' about her-eeee." When you're sitting there trying to go, why do you jump a foot off the seat when someone knocks on the door? Why do you frantically say "Busyyyy!!" or "Occupiedddd!!" like they don't know what you're doing. Why do dogs turn their head and look at you when they're pooping? Because their ass is hanging out for everyone to see and it's supposed to be private!

So, here's the deal. Nurses don't have all flippin' day to ask you about your bowel movements in a mild manner like, "So, what have you been doing all morning, hmmm? Reading or watching some fun TV show?" Or, "Take any trips somewhere else in the room today?" This might be a milder approach, but it ain't happenin'. It's funny, a nurse would never walk in and ask, "Did anyone come in this morning and stick a prong up your ass?" They wouldn't. They'd be all nice and use code words about it. But, when it comes to going to the bathroom, they're right there between the cheeks about it: "Time of movement?" "Color?" "Size?" "Elongated, ball shaped?" Come on!! I have no idea! #! Do I look like a person who checks!?

"Elongated" is a peculiar word because no matter when it's used, it's funny. Jackie and I visited Stratford-upon-Avon, England years ago, and while attending a tour of Shakespeare's home, an English woman with very large front teeth and really high gums led our tour. Pointing to a long, thick pole sticking out of a spire, Mrs. English Accent says, "As you can plaaainly see heeeearr…we haoovvv the eloooongatedddd pole of Sir Humphrey Gilbert." Jackie saw me holding back a laugh, and burst out laughing, putting her hand to her mouth so the guide wouldn't see who it was. The guide was so, so serious. "In 1638, this massive pole was used on ship Madeline's rigging; a fine vessel she was." We couldn't stop. Every time Jackie tried stifling another laugh, I would start up again. By the time the woman added more about "Sir Humphrey's elongated pole," it was useless. We had to slip out a side door!

In a relative matter, let me just say that men sometimes have a difficult time with elongation regarding female doctor checkups. You can scoff all you want, but controlling things down there is not as easy as women think. It can be intimidating. Things happen. Also, in your mind you're sure the doctor is going to lift up the front of your powder-blue gown, let cold air in, and say, in a Fargo accent, "Gee, pretty shriveled up there, aren't cha!"

The *Seinfeld* "Shrinkage" episode: It's just that male libidos seem to work differently than females', which is good actually, and just an observation from a guy and certainly not based on scientific fact. It's just that my maleness or whatever it is shows up whether I want it to or not. It's like back in fifth grade. Sometimes, totally out of the blue, things would happen down there. If you got a boner in history class at the end of the hour, you had to awkwardly hold your bookbinder in front of your pants walking out. You knew damn well Gloria would be walking next to you, wondering why your pants had a strange bulge doing the stick-out.

Females can feel free to write me regarding their side of the above and I'll see if we can get this book reprinted. Females probably have far more to say about this topic, but I can only speak for myself.

During my first lung transplant test at MMHMMM, a couple of female nurses came in and said they had a "poqiwnrasnfklwjqer" test to perform. I didn't even ask. All of a sudden one of them flung open the front of my blue gown and headed down U.S. 80 towards my groin and what now probably looked like a pink slinky toy. I was like, *Whoa, ahhhhh...so, ahhhhh…whoa...hey?!!* A pink slinky toy probably isn't the best way to describe what they were looking at because it changes as you go. I mean, it depends: warm air, cold air, thoughts. Maybe Thomas the Toy Train?

One of the nurses chuckled and said, "Don't worry, hon, what ya got goin' on be all the same plumbing!"

I never considered I had "plumbing goin' on." Ol' Coney down below immediately got offended and pulled even further inward, making him/it look like a doorknob.

Anyway, because you're going to be visited by 2,133 doctors in one week, you need to know the skinny about how it goes when you're in the doctor's office. Also, the doctor entrance thing:

First, doctors, nurses, whomever (if they have a hospital official emblem) may walk in and ask you to take your clothes off. It's not like this happens to you all the time in life—maybe it does—but... regardless, at some point, you'll have to get over it. It took a few times with me, but it's like you're in the zoo—someone is going to look.

Second, there's this thing with doctors'/PAs' clipboards. If a doctor/PA walks in without a clipboard and with their hands in the side pockets of their white lab coat, you are dealing with a very laid back, easygoing human. They will smile a lot, greet you with something creative like "How's it hanging?" (just kidding), or "Looks like you're up and at 'em"; "Sunny day, fun day"; something of that ilk. You can let your guard down with them, tell them a joke. They'll enjoy it and actually conjure up a laugh.

If the doctor/PA/intern walks in with a clipboard in hand, they'll be all business. Immediately they'll say, "Date of birth?" They don't mess with chat. They're all, "I've got 203 patients to visit today—you're number six, so..." Check, check, check...macaroni.

If the doctor/PA/intern walks in holding a clipboard tightly up by their neck with two hands, walks in short, chippy steps, hasn't had sex in three months, and has an unruly dog at home, you're in for it. Cold stethoscope, no chat, make it snappy questions like: "Name, birth, blood, tire pressure?" and the famous "Bowel movement?"

Here's info you need to know: Figure out who you're dealing with. Get to know your nurses, be nice to them, and continually remember: Nurses get a million questions a day, so think it over before looking out your window and saying, "Is it sunny out there?" Realize nurses have to answer you. They can't just stare at you like Dawn of the Dead. Sometimes they make like they don't hear you, which is understandable. But, like the highway road crews, "Giv'm a break!"

Because it's their job, sooner or later nurses have to answer questions like, "How does this phone work?" "What's that tube over there for?" or "Where does that catheter go again?" It's probably really hard for a staff person to keep from being majorly sarcastic. I'm sure they'd like to answer, "Like any other phone, dumbass," or "Let's see, where wouldddd a bladder catheter go, hmmm?"

And, more info. When you're in the hospital feeling like shit, depressed, bored, or teething, you start talking to anyone who is around. Anyone is fair game: staff, the janitor, the little old lady turtling by with her walker.

You do this because, one: Daytime TV sucks. Two: Asking questions takes your mind off how crappy you feel—and—three: You need someone to get you to the bathroom.

I wonder. Since staff members get so many questions all day, when they go to lunch and someone asks, "Where's the salt?"—bam!—they scream, "Right in front of your stupid, dumbass face!" I mean, they've got to get even at some point. When staff members go home at night and their kid asks, "Where do babies come from?" they probably duct tape 'em to the wall!

(BTW—It's "duct tape," not "duck tape." Not for taping ducks.)

Hospital work is tough. Looking at it from the staff's point of view is pretty interesting. Here're some thoughts I picked up from the staff:

The Tattoo / Missing Teeth Ratio

Evidently, hospital staff have figured out if a patient has over three tattoos and two or more missing teeth, said patient is going to be trouble, have a gun, and will sign hospital forms with an "X."

I'm sorry, I'm just repeating exactly what they told me. Not all patients come in sweet little packages like Pollyanna. You may think this is rude to say, but the fact is some people have never owned a toothbrush, haven't taken a shower/bath since President Carter, and believe every word radio shock jocks tell them. Medical staff put up with more than we ever want to know.

Families

We all like families. It's the family unit—the family picnic. Well, sometimes for good and fair reasons some families get whacky, especially around hospitals. We're talking out-of-control whacky. Not always, but hospital personnel will tell you, family matters are one of their worst nightmares. One staff person told me he came into a patient's room only to find a family member choking his brother. Just an average day on the job. They called security.

Be Proactive (I'm not talking about yogurt.)

Be totally proactive with every single thing that happens to you. This is paramount. MMHMMM offered great care, yet things still came up where, if I hadn't said something, it would have been bad. Hospitals and their medical personnel cannot be perfect allll the time. Their job and the place where they work are enormous and often unruly, busy, and damn complicated. I don't know how they get through half a day. Be on your toes. Same with your support group.

Ok, true story (which doesn't mean other stories have been fake). Heading into a pretty invasive procedure one day, my nurse was making sure things were in order, like they do. She was checking off the usual—date of birth, address, next of kin (that one always makes me nervous), type of car, favorite Beanie Baby, etc., when I asked her an important question. Hated to bother her, she had work to do, but something didn't seem right. After asking my "didn't seem right" question, the nurse gave me a slow, blank look, didn't say anything, and abruptly left the room.

Without going into finer detail, suffice to say the same nurse came back about ten minutes later and said, "Ahhh…Mr. Emmet, your surgery for this morning has been cancelled." From Ms. Chekov's stern expression, finding out what caused this quick change of heart was not going to happen. She said, with no attempt at an explanation, "They can't do surgery on you today. Sorry," clamped down her clipboard, and said, walking out the door, "Mary will help gather your things and set up a new surgery appointment." Something somewhere changed after I asked my one insignificant question.

I immediately commented as nicely as I could, "I got up at five thirty this morning, fought traffic for an hour, tried to find a place to park downtown, and arrived precisely at six thirty for this procedure.

Now, out of the blue, it's been called off?" Another blank look and pull of the curtain.

Yep, happened. The point is, speaking up was crucial. Had I not said something, I might have been in the middle of some surgical procedure with a doctor saying, "Nurse, this patient's chart says, 'Tire rotation'?" It was the old "needless to say" cliché. The whole debacle did notttt make my morning.

Later on, I found out my question was extremely significant. I was on blood thinners and no one had informed the surgical staff. Mistakes happen and avoiding them, no matter who is involved or whose feeling are hurt, is part of your survival. That sounds so dramatic, but you're not at a cider mill buying doughnuts. You're involved in serious situations and everyone knows it. This is no time to go, "Yeah, well, my IV has been squirting out some yellow stuff for the last hour, but I didn't want to say anything."

Ask questions and speak up. This is one time in your life it's ok. Everything around you is going to be new, foreign, and strange. Try to keep it from overwhelming you. Not easy, I know. If you go to the bathroom and what comes out glows and looks radioactive, make a fuss!

Then there's the following directions thing. As you saw with the wire in my nose and throat, following directions was difficult for me. If a doctor or staff member tells you to do something, you should do it—but only to a point. The following happened to me. I'm not making this up:

A physical therapist came in my room around the fifth or sixth day after my double-lung transplant surgery. She was a short, young woman full of energy. Ms. Bouncy had blond cropped hair, strong arms, and bangs. For some reason, she seemed sort of strangely beaming or wired. You know, the cartoon eyeballs coming too far out of their sockets look. Subsequently, I sensed I was either her first patient appointment after graduating with a 4.0 from her master's degree program, or she just downed two Starbucks triple expressos. There was just something way overboard going on with her.

Here I was, fresh meat from surgery. The word fresh is used here as in "fresh as an overly ripe tomato" or "a really dark brown avocado." Fragile. I was the patient who could be bruised if breathed on, or the one where the doctor said, "Sewing him up was like suturing Jell-O" kind of fresh. I was also higher than a kite from major meds. I know, you're thinking maybe this didn't happen because I was so drugged up, but, believe me, it did.

So, this brand spanking new (whatever that means ?) physical therapist arrives all powered up and ready to play! She told me her name was Poppy and she was excited because we were going to start doing our exercises!! (Take note of the exclamation points and words "we" and "our".) Whatttt exercises? Opening my eyes took effort, so there's that. I'm breathing up and down, which counts for my reps. Hmmm, I totally understood having to move in some way—emphasis on "some." Yes, immediately after surgery, or ASAP, you need to move so your body doesn't seize up. I get it. But when it comes to a double-lung transplant and certain situations—like mine!—"movin' ain't happenin'." Nada, nope, no way, discussion over.

I'm thinkin' ix-nay with the exercise-ay. Unfortunately, Ms. Bouncy Pants is sitting at the end of my bed with a big grin on her face. It wasn't a grin like Chucky, because, overall, she looked kindly, but there was something sinister in there. In a sort of screechy, excited voice, Ms. Bouncy told me to put my arms up above my head three times as quickly as possible. With goldfish eyes, I said, "Can't do that."

She came back with, "Sure you can! Wacko socko—we can make this happen!!" She was like my own personal spin instructor on crack.

My response was immediate, "Wacko socko—thatttt's not happenin'."

She came right back with, "Yessss it issss! That's what I'm here for!! Cutie. You're a tough guy. Come on!"

Looking straight down her throat to her tonsils, I said, "Look. I appreciate your help, but putting my arms above my head at this juncture is, in Spanish, 'Ni de coña.' Four days ago, surgeons practically cut me in half, which is not hyperbole. I have 227 stitches running from my left armpit, across my entire chest, to my right armpit. My sternum was cut in half. Not bruised: cut in half. Thinking about breathing hurts, let alone moving. Lifting my hand an inch off the bed might be a good start, so what you're asking is, pardon my French, out of the ——ing question."

All fired up like a Texas cheerleader on Beaver Buzz, the young PT said, "Come onnnn!! Yessss, you cannnn!!" tilting her head sideways and holding out the "yes" like she was feeding a six-month-old.

I came back with the same head tilt, "Noooo, I can'tttt!! Look!! Who sent you in here?" trying to be fairly decent, but getting more agitated.

She said, "I know, I know, but this will be gooood for you." Then, all of a sudden, Gidget started climbing up on the side of my bed.

I am not kidding!! I was like WTF! She quickly squeezed in behind me and said, "Here. Let me help!"

I was like, "Hey!!" but nothing was stopping her. I glanced at the door to see if a nurse was going by and could help me. She started trying to get a grip under my arms!!

I yelled for all I was worth, "Heyyyy!! Waa....Heyyyy!!"

Poppy said, "You can do it!!" I couldn't believe what was happening! And, I won't tell you what I screamed then. It was bad. Really bad. I went into Neanderthal mode. The volume of sound coming out of my mouth was heard two floors below. I couldn't do anything but yell. Two nurses came running in the room yelling, "Code Red! Code Red!" Then I passed out.

When I came to, they told me what happened. I must have really scared—or scarred—the shit outta Poppy...a.k.a. Dick the Bruiser. Ms. Bouncy had fallen off the bed onto the hospital floor, and staff were in the room yelling.

Gaining my wits, I said in a loud voice, "WTF!? Mother Teresa over there tried to kill me! @#!" I was still angry and yelled, "What in hell were you thinking!!" holding on to my chest with both arms so everything inside wouldn't come shooting out. "Are you ——ing nuts! @#! I'm cut in half and you try that !@#"

One male nurse was hovering over me like I was going to attack, which obviously wasn't going to happen. Another nurse ushered the now-dazed, first-day physical therapist out the door. Her blond hair was all messed up, her PT badge upside down, and she was saying something about not telling her supervisor.

"See me...feel me...touch me..." from the Who's *Tommy* album only goes so far.

Make changes when necessary.

This is another important item on the list. Understand you and your support group have a say in things. You know, like what's going to happen to you next. Incidents happen, even at Resort Day at Hospital Beach. One afternoon a rookie nurse was prepping me for an IV. Overseeing her was a garrulous old nurse who looked like she had given one too many enemas and seemed very, very disinterested. Baby Nurse with bangs, standing about five feet, maybe, and looking way too young to be poking my arm with anything, let alone a sharp needle, was obviously going to try to find a vein and get my IV going. She said, "Ok, let's see...um...First I'm supposed to set out a plastic bag with the needle in it on the tray." I sensed, after experiencing hundreds of these innocent pokes for innocent IVs, this wasn't starting off well. Sort of a "she's reading directions" thing.

With needle pack on tray, Ms. Trainee said in a kid's voice, "I'm now going to get your IV started," while strapping the proverbial rubber band around my bicep. "It's gonna sting like an itty-bitty bee." I should have stopped the whole procedure on "itty-bitty," but thought she needed a chance. After all, how do trainees train, right? She fumbled around getting the needle out of the wrong end of the plastic package that read "open here" at the top, which gave me all sorts of confidence. Then, she started slapping/snapping the skin on the inside of my elbow...like they all do.

At some point, Ms. Trainee said, "I'm going in now," in a shaky voice. "Hope it doesn't hurt."

Time out...Let me explain something before we go on. Having a needle go into your skin isn't so bad if it's one of those skinny ones. I found out they have these very small-in-diameter needles for jobs such as this. They do make big bazooka needles for some applications I don't want to know about. Anyway, where the trouble shows up is when the nurse gets said needle in your arm, but can't find the vein they "thought" was "right there." It's like someone using a GPS who can't figure out where to turn. What happens next is not—I repeat—not good. The nurse can't find the vein, gets shaken, nervous, upset, withdrawn, depressed, and gets a Howdy Doody look on her face. She says, "I don't know what's the matter; I know it's in there somewhere ...??." Oh, damn.

Then, yow!...sting!…and now, with the needle in my arm, Miss Pre-teen USA starts doing what I call the "needle hokey pokey." This, as you know all too well if you've ever gotten more than one IV, is where they can't find the vein they're looking for and commence moving said needle around inside to "find it." Double damn.

Pulling the needle back out would seem to be the humane thing to do in this disturbing situation, but they're driven. They're totally sure it's "right there." They're on a mission to find that sucker. In truth, they need to go to lunch, get a Starbucks coffee, or maybe go to the bathroom. But "nooo." By God, they're going to find it. After three or four tries left, right, behind, and through every nerve inside your arm, they give up and say, "Let's try another spot, ok?" Was that a question? Like can I say, "No. It's my football; I'm going home." Evidently, said IV was necessary for my upcoming procedure so there was no option. What happens next is, as you probably guessed—try, try again.

Once you're on this stick'em Merry-Go-Round, a wise choice is to ask for someone higher up the needle-wielding ladder. I mean it. You'll regret it if you don't. I didn't this time, trying to be nice and all. Of course, now we're heading into a radish patch of attempts. On the fifth and unsuccessful stabbing, exploring, and takin' a look-see, Goldilocks says, cracking her gum, "Ya know, I'm not having a very good day."

At that point, with my arm now resembling a pincushion, I said, "Ya know, I'm not either."

Turning to the older head nurse in the room who looked like she justttt might be a tiny bit better at the needle deal, I said, "I'm not trying to be difficult, but could we get someone else to do this IV?" Not wanting to make the young trainee cry, I started softly singing in falsetto voice the Supremes's "Some days there are days like this, days like this someeee times." I always try to divert when I'm about to use really bad swear words. The head nurse slowly ambled over like it was the long road to China and said, "Sweetie, y'all go on, I'll take care of this one," like I was the next pig in line at the meat plant. Goldie ran out of the room upset and with her head downcast.

My head was downcast for a much different reason. My arm hurt—a lot. Without saying a word and without letting me get a complaint in edgewise, the Judy Dench look-alike grabs my hand and snaps the top of it really hard. That spot was getting mighty sore, but evidently there was a vein yelling, "Slap me! Pick me!" and she inserted a needle. Immediately, to my relief, blood started running. My blood. It followed the tube up to my IV bag, and Ms. Head Nurse secured whatever and walked back to what she was doing. Bim-bam-done. Silence. As I started to say something, Head Nurse turned and said, "She's a rookie. She'll learn."

I was really happy my arm was available for training purposes.

Side note: I did have a very unfortunate incident happen to me whilst in the hospital and I am bringing it up only because it drives home the "make changes if needed—speak up" theme. To say it was a bad moment at an extremely difficult time for me would be an understatement. Suffice to say, what happened didn't go well when it really needed to go well. It was the most difficult moment of my entire lung transplant experience and one that still haunts me.

I didn't want to mention this confrontation, because my stay and surgery at MMHMMM was extraordinary and went unbelievably well. I just want you to understand speaking up, not putting up, needs to be part of your thought process and your family's as well. Some of the time you'll be in La La Land from your meds and won't be able to make decisions for yourself. Therefore, it's essential your family/support group is fully aware they too need to speak up if and when a situation arises. If someone doesn't, the hospital staff might not be aware. Doctors and nurses don't have crystal balls and can't be by your side every second. There were quite a few times when Kristen or Dr. Anisee said, "If something happens, tell us. Don't keep it to yourself. That's why we're here. We don't want to know something after the fact."

As with most things, reacting and speaking up is a balancing act. You can't go overboard because that can screw things up in the opposite direction. We've all met someone here or there who, when given the chance, can make a mountain out of a small ant hill or take a normal situation and blow it sky high. (I know you're thinking of exactly who that might be right now. You are, I know you are.) Some people purposely give others a hard time or make things overly dramatic. Some pick on waitstaff, some just like to make a scene. People who act this way seek attention, but that's another circus. When I mention speaking up, I'm not referring to being overly picky or complaining just to complain. I'm referring to things like if they incorrectly wrote, "Cut this one —>" on the wrong leg.

Regarding my particular incident, I spoke up. I had to. I told my lung transplant team what happened and it was immediately dealt with. No organization can employ perfect people and it would be ridiculous to expect perfection from any large group of individuals. We all try, but, in the end, we're human, not robots. Sometimes we make mistakes. Taken all and all, I tried to put this incident behind me.

Never be bullied into something you know is wrong. Unless it's an immediate emergency, there's time to make sure things are correct. It's not like everyone's got a hot date or a plane to catch. If you ask a question and find out everything's fine, great. At least you spoke up. It shows you're on it and being proactive. If you tell someone your nurse just threw a large elephant out your seventh-floor window, they'll know your narcotics are in full bloom and will pantomime sweeping up the broken glass for you.

Throughout my life, whenever something bad happened to my body, I knew it. When I was young, I broke my arm playing baseball. At the local hospital, a young intern felt it and said, "Don't worry; your arm's fine, not broken." I knew it was broken. I could feel it. After an x-ray, the same intern walked back in my room and said rather flippantly, "Yeah, it's broken."

Listen to your body; it talks to you more than you would think.

Ok, more suggestions. Thank your staff each and every time things go right. Do not thank them when something goes wrong because they'll think you're being a smart ass. As in, "Thanks so much for missing my vein for the seventh time!" Do not say that.

Believe me, once you've been in a hospital awhile, you soon realize how exceedingly complicated it is to run 52,357,107 floors chock full of the wildest equipment the likes of which you have never seen. And, that's just the machines, scans, screens, probes, ceiling fans, bedpans, wires, monitors, and miles and miles of tubes. Did you ever see the movie *Brazil*? Google it—we're talkin' tubes and tubes. It's like Willy Wonka's chocolate factory on crack. And, we're only covering hardware. When you add the human element to the physical plant, holy schnnnikies! Ten million staff people whizzing around trying to do everything under the sun! That is to say, "let me count the ways." Whomever is in charge—wow! Impressive! Hospitals are mountainous.

When you sit back and consider the breadth of it all, a hospital's complexity is vast and remarkable. But you also realize, if you boil all of it down to its base, individual human beans make it all work, make it go. All the machines in the world can't make impromptu decisions on life or death at the exact second needed, can't untangle thirty-three wires just before they explode, can't serve breakfast with a real smile, and, importantly, can't deeply care.

Maybe future hospitals will run themselves. I don't think it will be soon though, seeing as self-driving cars are doing so well. Maybe 3037? I don't know. I'll be 1,019 years old, so "ehhh." I'll be a skeleton going into a bar ordering a beer and a mop. But, as of now, it's the staff. They're the ones. The staff helped me get through many overwhelming trials. And, I really did thank them every—single—time.

During my stay at MMHMMM, I also found saying something positive to a staff member means more to them than you think. I told one doctor she was amazing, because she was, and her work meant more to me than she would ever know. It was a bit wordy and not very eloquent, but it was all I could think of to say. What she said back surprised me: "Thank you, that really means a whole lot to me." It seemed like she wasn't used to being thanked. How could anyone have their life changed or saved without thanking the one who made it happen—over and over and over. Tell the person making your bed, "Thank you." Old fashioned, no. The right thing to do, yes.

Exercise your ass off. Be top of your rock-climbing team, your bridge club, parachute gang, or ping-pong pals. Be Lance Armstrong, minus the steroids, be LeBron James soaring above the rim. If you're even younger yet, just exercise and shut up.

We all talk about exercising, but few actually do it consistently. "Yep, I swim twenty laps a day!" In truth, it was probably only one lap to the poolside bar. We all embellish our workouts because it's fun and it sounds so good, but I'm telling you from experience, if you are strong going into intense and difficult procedures, you'll do so much better when you come out the other side. The moment you try to start moving around, your prior strength will truly help.

I made a plan to exercise the areas/muscles needed the most in my recovery. First and foremost was my right forearm to my mouth. Just kidding, but not. I really got that ol' chip-to-dip to movement down to a science. Of course, I made that my first goal! Whether they told me drinking beer was ok or not, some items not to be named were going to be lifted with those specific arm muscles (beer), and I knew (beer) said muscles (beer) had to be toned and ready.

I know, I know, I shouldn't joke about any of this. In fact, if I truly shouldn't, this whole book should be banned, like people tried to do with my high-school teaching copy of *Catcher in the Rye*.

Anyway, my plan was to do ten squats and ten pushing myself up and out of a chair right before each meal—breakfast, lunch, and dinner. Since missing a normal meal never happened, this plan would always remind me to do these fun squats and pushes. Sounds like English pub food—Squats & Pushes w/ Bangers & Ma*s*h, followed by a pint.

Find a place away from people, squat down, and stand back up ten times. Then find a chair, sit down and then push up from the chair with only your arms, holding your legs off the floor. Up the repetitions as you get stronger. Get your legs with squats, and arms and shoulders with the chair thing.

These particular moves were only done at home. Restaurants, dinner parties, and business after hours' appetizer gatherings were exempt, even though bathrooms worked, back hallways, anywhere to keep from appearing completely whacked. But you can't give in. No excuses.

Take a really close look at what's going to happen to your body when you go through surgery. Google it. It's there, believe me, camera closeups and all, the whole enchilada. You can watch the whole thing. Pinpoint the muscle groups you'll need the most. It's not rocket science. Actually, your PT will show you everything. Then, just do it. Do it whether you want to or not. Do it before every meal, or don't eat. I'm telling you, you have to get durable and strong, or you'll pay dearly later.

Did I do them every single day? No.

Come on, how many of us follow a strict plan for health reasons? "January first, I'm going to start on my diet." That's like Custer saying, "Don't worry, we've got plenty of men." Sure, I missed a few days here and there. But I'll have to say, I kept at it, tried hard not to skip days, and eventually got much, much stronger. "Before your surgery" is the key phrase. This has to happen before.

Find ways to strengthen your core. A good friend of mine is an occupational therapist and while I was a "pre," she encouraged me to work on my core. Core: the area between waist and neck—sort of. She still insists it's the most important area of all. She's right.

Do you have to be a fanatic about it? Fanatics get up at five a.m. for morning runs in rain, snow, and slush; work out in smelly, grimy gyms incessantly; make healthy smoothie drinks from things like spinach, grass, fish juice, tabasco, kale, cardboard, and, my favorite, wheat germ mixed with raw eggs. They lift weights so heavy it takes two huge strangers to get the barbell back on the rack. I mean, more power to them, but you're probably notttt going to do anything close.

It's just that most of us try a plan. A week later we're like, "What plan? Was there a plan?" If I wasn't so consistently non-consistent, some of my plans might have worked. But this was different. There was going to be a surgery. My body was taking part in that surgery. It was going to happen. There comes a time where "yeah, maybe" has to become a must. What you're headed into isn't something lighthearted. This is the real deal. You are going to need strength—badly. To be fair, I did do the squats and pushes more than you might think. A lot was accomplished, and it helped me greatly post-surgery trying to get up from a toilet or scamper out of bed. Alright, "scamper" is hyperbole...but I like the sound of it. Makes me sound like a light, speedy chipmunk, which is so far from the way I was, it's ridiculous. Truth—after my surgery, I was a sloth. When Jackie and Zachera went to the Lincoln Park Zoo one day, they brought a stuffed animal sloth to be my hospital buddy. I called him Sloth.

Another major suggestion from the ol' experience notebook, and one that helped immensely, is: After having a double-lung transplant or recovering from any massive health issue, take each day one day at a time. Old clichés linger, but they are still around. Why? Because they are true. Following clichés like "one day at a time" will help you—I promise. When you're involved in a serious procedure, it's easy to get caught up with tomorrow, next week, next month. You're involved in something too big to think that far ahead. Keep a tight hold on today.

I've never, ever been remotely small, slight, light, or svelte. I am (was) a six feet two, 230-pound linebacker type. People like me call ourselves big boned. When I was born, the nurse said, "Forget the bassinet; get a refrigerator box." Therefore, trying to get myself off a hospital bed after surgery was equivalent to a water buffalo trying to get out of a deep, mucky hole. Not easy, took lots of work.

Side point: I came out of my transplant shy of six feet. I shrunk. Nobody told me why, and I didn't ask because the answer is probably scary.

Anyway, one fairly blank, boring day, I was alone in my hospital room and came up with the interesting idea of trying to get to the bathroom by myself. Hadn't accomplished this yet, and performing that procedure in a bedpan made my Top Ten Most Uncomfortable, Messy, Irritating Life Experiences List. Ok, at least guys have a spigot. I can't speak for women. In fact, I don't get their deal at allll when it comes to that. Regardless, male or female, the second movement of the "Bathroom Suite" by Charmin is impossible to do in a bedpan. Not going into the details, but pretty impossible. Add in stitches, broken bones, bloated stomachs, and what all—you've got nothin' but nasty. Because of this, I was highly motivated to make it to my room's bathroom. Of course, said bathroom was on the other side of my room's Grand Canyon. Taking one singular move at a time, it could be done. Might take two hours, but it was a challenge and beat watching old reruns of *Wheel of Fortune*.

After about twenty minutes, I had one leg on the floor and one leg still stuck under the covers. All my tubes were tangled and one fell out. At that point, it wasn't going to happen, which, one: was a bladder/bowel problem, and, two: was a "I can't stay in this position very long, because circulation to my lower extremities will soon cease" problem. Luckily, Shipshawnna came by my room to take my lunch order.

Ship took one look and came right over to my bedside. "Wat you doin'! Y'all trying ta git out the bed!! Iiii tole you, don't, cause y'all be hurtin'," she exclaimed. "Naw I got git you right, an fo' sure I got betta thangssss to doooo!" She went on and on like that "givin' me hell." I deserved it and loved it at the same time because I knew Ship cared. She always tried to make me comfortable no matter what it took. We laughed together, and a few times cried together.

Shipshawnna saved my ass quite a few times during my stay, and talking with her always made me smile. Her sing-song vernacular, her hearty, 290-pound (?) laugh, deep and full, made difficult moments ok. I loved her no-nonsense attitude. When I was constipated, she'd stand outside my bathroom door and say, "Just do it, fooo." I think she made me laugh so hard I finally did go!

Ship kidded me a lot, but she was trying to help. I wasn't in a "good place," as they say, and she did whatever she could to lessen the angst. She probably didn't know how much she meant to her patients. It's hard to put down in words what someone like Ship means when you're sick or hurt. As we move through life, it's the little things that count the most. Funny how one individual can make such a difference.

Years ago, I attended a beautiful funeral service for a beautiful friend who died from cancer. Her name was Catherine. She was a tall, dark-haired woman with deep eyes and an almost haunting look. It was as if she was every ethnic group in the world, all in one. Catherine was extremely educated and smart. She was one of those people you meet that just sort of "know."

Catherine knew she was dying for a long time and recognized the end when it came. She left her family a recording to be played during her memorial. When they played it in the small church across from her house, it was so wonderful to hear her voice again—albeit strange in the given setting. What she said never left me, "It's the little things that mean the most. Walking down my front sidewalk to get the morning's mail, sitting at my kitchen table sipping a cup of just brewed coffee, tending my flowers. It's not the big things. It's the small moments."

She asked us to savor them as we go along our way.

I have ever since. As I said in the beginning of this book, it's moments. After having someone donate their loved one's lungs to me and having gifted doctors let me breathe again, Catherine's words ring in my mind and heart every single day.

15

Lots of Plants

People come up to me in my small hometown and say, "I heard about your lung transplant. I didn't even know they could do that!" The funny thing is, so many make the same comment, yet, surprisingly, there are all these other human beans who say, "Oh, yeah, a lung transplant. My Uncle Erv got that done last year, and they're lookin' at that as a possibility for my neighbor down our street, too. I'm gettin' a breast reduction next month cause I'm tired of these babies gettin' in the way all the damn time!" She said all this like everyone just walked down to the farmer's market, bought some strawberries, lettuce, grabbed a lung transplant, and walked home. Pretty wild.

True story: I was sitting in our little town's Boyne City Bakery one day—a wonderful French bakery run by exceedingly friendly and talented owners. A small group of our friends met there on Tuesdays, but on this particular day I was alone. A man I didn't know came in and got a coffee and croissant. He sat down at a table across from mine and said, "Damn hot out there!"

I answered, "I know! Hot for up here! Northern Michigan isn't normally this warm and muggy."

Since we were both alone, we struck up a conversation. He was an elderly man in old fashioned pleated pants with suspenders. What hair he had left looked like it had once been a brush cut

(Google if you're younger than fifty). After talking for a few minutes, he said, "Up visitin' my granddaughter; she been sick."

I immediately said, "Ah, that's too bad. She going to be ok?"

He said something back that floored me, "She been sick with breathin' and such. Got herself one of those lung transplants, I think they call it."

This man was a complete stranger. Such a coincidence. But little did I know what he was going to say next. Before I could tell him I had just gone through the exact same unbelievable transplant, he went on, "Damn tough girl that Shelly is. The first transplant didn't take after the first eight months or so. Somethin' about immune something. Reject somethin', I think she called it."

Butting in, I said, "Holly cowwww," which was a really dumb thing to say, but I couldn't come up with anything else. What he was saying was crazy. At first, from what he said I thought she must have died. What do you say to that? But then he said he was "up visitin'." Did he mean he was visiting her kids or husband?

"Shelly, she been in the hospital a lot. Like I say, she's a tough one. When the first set of them lungs didn't work, they sent her back to get two more! Two new ones! Now she's up and bossin' ever one around."

"What? She got another lung transplant after the first one?!" I said.

"Yep, Shelly said they told her she's one of the very few in the country who's done it twice. Said was cuz she's so young and strong, you know. I said to her, 'Shelly, you means if your new ones blow, ya get a third set?!' Shelly slapped her knee sittin' there and said, 'Damn straight I am, Grandpa!' We laughed at that; we did!"

After our conversation ended and the older gentleman went on his way, I walked outside the little bakery in a daze. Standing there in the morning sun, I thought, "What in the world am I going to hear next?" I don't know. It's just weird. The whole transplant thing is strange, bizarre, futuristic, and getting my head around it still hasn't happened. Transplanting hearts, kidneys, livers, pancreases, hips, thumbs, or brains is the stuff of Mr. Doud's science class's little "The Future" newsletter and its hovercraft cars.

Ok, they don't do brains—yet—but you know they will. The problem with transplanting brains is…who the hell are you afterward? That's what's holding them back on the brain thing. You got to be you. I mean, I like Coney dogs, but what if my new brain doesn't?! And, another thing, once they transplant your brain, do they call you Jim or the other guy? Maybe you're a third guy? I don't know.

The whole spectrum of public understanding when it comes to modern medicine goes from those who have never heard of these unbelievable feats of surgery to those who take them as commonplace. This spectrum is a vast, open arena full of people understanding, misunderstanding, and being oblivious. No matter how people view transplants or any of the myriad astounding medical advances today, none—and I mean none—of it is mundane or commonplace. Yes, these surgeries are being performed daily. They're still inconceivable, though. The medical field is creating new and fantastic ways to keep us alive, trying to give us a good quality of life. To me, all of these feats of science and medicine will always be a giant wonder.

All sorts of organs, parts, and darts are now on the grocery list. Hips and knees are big this year. For instance, I have two lungs from another human being, two new plastic lenses in my eyes giving me 20/20 vision, and take twenty-two pills a day to suppress my immune system so it won't attack my new lungs like Attila the Hun. Sometimes I picture all my pill chemicals gathering like a biker gang near my lungs, fighting and diverting those immune system guys. "Hey, munies, over here! Ignore those two lungs. Catch us if you can!" they yell as they pull wheelies and head out toward my thalamus. I don't know.

Doctors have opened up my knee, shoulder, eyes, arm, explored my arteries via a wire up my groin, stayed in Vegas overnight, and sped down Route 66 into my heart—check, check, check. They've sewed things up, scratched around, filed, plucked, and attached things until I was right again. Most important of all, my doctors somehow took my lungs out and then put someone else's lungs in. A handshake and a smile later, they sent me on my way. Now that is pretty damn amazing. More amazing than words can convey.

As things go, it's always interesting how one gets from one place or another in life. I mean, how you ended up here, or there. What cosmic force kept you from stepping in front of that speeding car? How did you happen to meet the one you love out of hundreds of thousands? I'm not sure there's an answer.

Whilst younger, I played football, baseball, soccer, basketball, and was insane enough to play rugby in college, which is ten times more dangerous than football and played without padding, helmet, or a brain. During my first rugby game for MSU's rugby club, we played Notre Dame. One of our forwards ran off the field screaming, "Doc! Doc!"

Our trainer shouted, "Mav, what ya got?!"

Maverick replied, "Ahhhh, damn shoulder popped out! Ahhhh!!"

The trainer grabbed a towel, swirled it into a rope, threw it over Mav's neck and under his arm, and yanked violently, forcing Mav's arm back into his shoulder socket. Mav screamed holy hell and then said in a calm voice, "Thanks Doc, ya got it," and immediately ran back into the game. That was rugby.

In my first scrum that day, the referee whistled, "scrum"—which is sort of like a huddle with everyone on the field locking shoulders, pushing, and poking each other in the eye. Whilst we were tugging, pushing, poking, and swearing, the Notre Dame player across from me slugged me in the mouth. Since the referee was standing right next to me, I yelled, "Hey, what the hell, he just punched me!"

The referee yelled back, "Playyyy rugbyyyy!" Ahhhh, so that's it!?! I punched the guy back, and on it went like that for the whole game. After watching this bloody medieval battle, my dad drove home and purchased more health insurance.

But, as things go, playing rugby at MSU led me somewhere else in life. How the hell does that happen? How does anything lead you somewhere? I don't know, but it does. It's not a question of whether it does or doesn't, it's a question of how and where. Makes no sense, but if you're reading this as a human being, you know exactly what I'm talking about.

My life's been quite a journey. For real—I've been hiking; camping; biking; sailing; swimming; canoeing; mud wrestling (very weird); I ran a half triathlon; ran the full Detroit Marathon under the Detroit River; played baseball in the Detroit Amateur Baseball Federation and pitched a game in Tiger Stadium (not Comerica); played broomball with a bunch of Polish butchers (literally) in Detroit's Eastern Market, then watched hotdogs being made (which you really don't want to do); won championships playing linebacker in football; ballooned over a Michael Jackson concert at the Palace in a, you guessed it, hot air balloon (long story); locked fifty live lobsters in the trunk of my car on a ninety-eight degree day (longer story); flew over the Grand Canyon in a helicopter and couldn't hear one damn word the guide said; rode a horse on the narrow and rocky cliffs of the Grand Tetons, which I highly recommend if you want a very short life; chased pigs (literally) on MSU's campus when they bolted loose from our animal husbandry class; and took part in panty raids—a college late-night ritual where hundreds and hundreds of guys chase parachuting size-fifty women's underwear sent flying from top dorm windows by lusty female coeds (no logical explanation).

All of this—and I mean all of it—wound a path to my next morning, my next day. You're in life's game, you line up, and hike the ball. What play do you run? How will it turn out? You're not sure, but at that very moment, right then, you're there.

In terms of your health, what you did to your body all those years is what doctors call "life accumulation." It's from doing crazy things but loving it, taking chances, making the mad blood flow, making life extraordinary. It's throwing acorns at each other from our bikes when we were ten, tobogganing down a steep, snowy path with my brother-in-law without knowing what loomed at the bottom, thus crashing our toboggan into a million pieces, wood everywhere. Mr. Toboggan's last ride. We laughed until we cried, and loved...loved...every second.

Through all of it—bumps, bruises, surgeries, scary moments, a near life-ending disease, heartaches, joy, headaches, wonderful experiences, sorrow, elation—I wouldn't change a thing. I've had a life. Still, though, the elephant in the room is, why was I so amazingly lucky? Everything lined up with my double-lung transplant, lucky at every turn. How does that happen?

Intertwined with this luck, phenomenal care, and support, were patients who underwent procedures and weren't so lucky. Things didn't work out. Some endured incredibly difficult days. When surgeries have to be redone due to infection, when doctors can't get all the tumor, when the cancer comes back, when heartache becomes a strongman pulling you deeper and deeper into despair, it takes a hero to keep going. I met many heroes whose recovery took months and months. Some ended in death.

What I witnessed and took special note of was how patients who had terribly difficult complications kept on keeping on. If a setback emerged, they got tougher and got through it. If another problem showed up, they went through the same awful thing again. Sometimes again and again. But they kept on keeping on.

One day, a year or two after my surgery, while visiting MMHMMM for my bi-monthly checkup, I heard someone hailing me from the middle of the hospital's vast general waiting area. It was Frank, with his smiling wife, Bonnie. Frank was in the room next to mine on the infamous seventh floor where most of the lung transplant patients hung out. We were both about the same age—our sixties—and had a lot in common. Frank had a double-lung transplant and a heart bypass at the same time, but there he was with Bonnie by his side. I walked over and gave them both a big hug.

Bonnie, a gal whose family had immigrated from Poland during the ravages of WW II, would smile her wonderful smile and say, "Frankie's doin' great! We're here for our checkup. You?" She said "our checkup" because she, just like Jackie, never left his side. Through all his difficult days, it was "we."

I answered, "Yep, 11:20 a.m...don't be late, right?"

Frank quipped, "They don't like it much if they call your name and you ain't there!"

Bonnie leaned in closer like she was telling a secret and laughingly whispered, "Frank's eating my kraut and Polish sausage and lovin' it, but we're not telling the lung team! They'd have a fit!!"

All three of us laughed out loud. I asked how things were going. Frank said, "Doin' betta. Can't complain. Damn site betta than before!" His heart was pumping strong, he looked great, and there wasn't an oxygen machine in sight!

All of the "posts" (as opposed to "pres") talk about "before." It is the metric—the measurement—of how we were before, and how we are now. Even those who had it really tough say "doin' betta than before." How incredible is it that someone arrives at the lung team's pulmonary-department door barely breathing and dying from diseased lungs, and then ... a year later ... tells me, with a robust smile, about how they're "doin betta." How can that be quantified?

16

The Visit

On a grey late afternoon, near the end of sixth day or so of my hospital testing stay, the head of MMHMMM's lung transplant team, Dr. Anisee, knocked on my hospital door and stepped in. "Care for a visitor?"

"A visit from you? Anytime," I smiled. "I feel privileged to see you this late. What's up?" I was telling the truth. It was quite surprising to see her walk in after the faint knock on the door. It had been a long, tedious round of tests that day and I guessed it probably had been even longer for her.

Dr. Anisee was my favorite person in the whole hospital. Yes, she was the head of the lung transplant team, one of the top programs in the United States, but you'd never know it by her demeanor. She was soft spoken to the point of quiet. She was five feet two, maybe, but had a presence that couldn't be explained. She was powerful in a very subtle way. You could feel it in the room—there was everyone else, and then there was her.

She was slender and diminutive, and had large dark Indian eyes that glistened. Whether with other patients, a nurse, or with me, she always smiled like she knew. I couldn't explain it. It was like she knew everything there was to know. Each time I said something to her, she understood, had guessed the nature of my comment, and seemed to know the best thing to say.

The day was waning, city lights were coming on, and snow was starting to fall. Dr. Anisee walked up close to me, next to the bay window. She had on a deep purple car coat, red leather gloves, dark heeled shoes, and was clutching a handbag matching her coat. Since it was evening, she was most likely heading home. We both looked out over the city and didn't say anything for a moment. I asked her if she'd like to sit down on the bay window's padded bench. She did, and looked at me through her wide, knowing eyes.

"It's late, why are you out and about visiting patients at this hour?" I asked.

"Nothing else to do," she laughed. She had a quick wit and was always upbeat. If there was anyone in the world who had nothing to do, it wasn't her.

"No, really?" A private visit without the rest of the team was rare, especially from Dr. Anisee, so I knew something was up.

She looked out the window again, as though she was quietly thinking. As it turned out, she was. She was thinking about me. I knew she was tired after another stressful day of decisions. She finally turned her soulful eyes to me and said, "I was headed home and thought I'd stop by so we could have a talk."

This didn't sound good—"thought I'd stop by" was one thing, but "have a talk," another. Negative thoughts popped into my head—*there was a test I didn't pass, they found something.* Of course, my tests always weighed heavily. If I didn't pass one, it was either get whatever they found fixed, or give up getting a lung transplant entirely. Heavy consequences. So, here was my head doctor—the head of everything in the world—saying she thought she'd stop by?

I had to be honest. "I'm so happy you took time to see me, but my guess is, this is more than chat. Kind of like when a teacher calls you up to their desk."

She shook her head. "Well…actually, I wanted to sit and talk with you to see how you were doing and what you were thinking."

Her comment still sounded serious. This wasn't normal conversation, even with Dr. Anisee. Up to this point, no one in the hospital had asked me what I was thinking, just: does this hurt? Can you tell me what year it is? Or—what do you want for lunch? There was just something about her words, but maybe it was nothing at all. It had been a stressful week of tests and I had to hold my breath each time the results showed up, hoping I would pass. The stakes were extremely high. I used to worry about flunking math in fifth grade. This was for a lot more marbles.

After rolling a million scenarios around in my head, I finally answered Dr. Anisee's "thoughts" question. "Well…ah…now that you ask…um…I've been thinking about a lot of things. I'm thinking a double-lung transplant is very big. Much bigger than I thought. Well, wayyyy bigger than I thought…ya know…big…and…" The same thoughts were coming out as those when Jackie, Zachera, and I talked that late night in the hotel room. It all came flowing out again. "I mean…ah…it's just…you don't think about these things until they actually happen, right…till they show up…ya know. I mean…at least I didn't. Now it seems all of a sudden I'm in the middle of life or death, a place I've never been, never imagined."

I paused, thinking I was talking too much and taking up Dr. Anisee's time. To my surprise, she quietly asked, "What else?"

"I…ah…well…been thinking about the fact that I'm getting worse, ya know. I mean I can feel it every day. So my thoughts are, what if I don't pass the last tests? What if the team finds something wrong and I never get donor lungs? All of you have been so kind to say if you found something serious, you'd just fix it, but I know, especially at my age, you're being hopeful for my sake and it's at best a maybe. There are some unfixable problems out there. I mean…if something's unfixable, the team wouldn't be able to put me on the donor list. There's just so much, so much to think about, to consider, so many variables. The process could take a long time—time I may not have. It's scary…way scary. Staying positive is important, but what if something goes wrong—that's it. There's no other road. If this doesn't work, I'm going to die soon."

I started to cry. It was quiet and I was embarrassed because it had happened once before with Dr. Anisee and the team when talking about my wonderful friends and Boyne City's special night to raise money for me. I didn't want Dr. Anisee to think this happed all the time. It all overwhelmed me again, just like it did with Jackie and Zachera. Having Dr. Anisee sitting in my hospital room put me at the pinnacle, the apex of the whole deal. Sitting next to me, she represented everything and much more, the future. She represented living or dying. This incredible, learned woman held my life in her hands.

She said, "I know this is all so much. It's hard to take in and it changes each day."

Trying to conceal the moisture around my eyes, I said, "It is. It's been such a rollercoaster ride already. Some days it seems like it's all going to work out and then there're too many variables, too many things that could go wrong, and I'll never get there. I'll die."

Dr. Anisee looked at me with her perceptive dark eyes. "Robert, there's a point where patients with IPF, COPD, and other lung diseases get so sick the chances of a healthy recovery from a lung transplant are very low. Our team tries to put an emphasis on listing patients who indeed need new lungs, but who are also strong and healthy. Patients healthy enough to go through the rigors of such a massive procedure and live through it."

Listening fixedly, I said, "That makes sense. I mean...I'm going downhill fast. It's strange though, because I don't feel weak. I'm strong. I can do things, you know, get around. I even try to work out almost every day. It's not easy, but I do. It's harder to breathe, but the thing is, I'm almost sixty-seven years old and your team said the cutoff point for admitting transplant patients is seventy. That doesn't give me much time even if my lungs level out some and don't get worse for a while."

With the same intensity, Dr. Anisee said, "You are declining faster than we first thought. The team went over your stats yesterday and it is very apparent your lungs are not the same as they were even just a few weeks ago. That seems to be how pulmonary fibrosis progresses—patients plateau for a few months and their stats level off, but then for no reason start to decline again. The problem is IPF never seems to go the other way, to get better. Patients may plateau, but when we first met you, the team thought you would be a possible future patient way down the road. As it turns out, that's not the case. Your intuitiveness regarding your body was correct. Your lung capacity is lessening, but you have strong health numbers in other aspects. Your tests prove that."

"The whole thing is closing in on me," I said quietly. Emotions were cresting inside.

"This is why I came to talk to you tonight. I wanted to see where your thoughts were," Dr. Anisee said.

We sat for a moment, not saying anything and looking out at the city lights. Dr. Anisee said, "I wanted to find out if you're ready— mentally. We know your physical test results, but needed to know where you were in terms of all this…inside."

I said, "I appreciate that more than you know."

"After all you've been through the last week or so, after all our talks in between, I think you're ready. You want to do this, don't you?" It was much more of a statement than a question.

I gave out a long sigh, a sigh that had been waiting inside me for a long time.

"I do. I so want to do this, to keep living. I'll do whatever it takes and make it work…if I can get the chance. Dr. Anisee, I'm not afraid to die. I never have been. There's never been a moment where I second guessed getting a transplant ever since Dr. Danzer introduced me to you and your team. I was kind of shocked at first. Then I started questioning my body's ability to pass all the tests. Sure, I worry about my family, but I worry for them—not me. I worry about my daughter's life—for her. I wonder what Jackie will do if I'm gone—but I worry for her, not me. None of it is for me. I've had my life and it's been extraordinary. I've never once looked over luck's shoulder. Wanting more in life would be absurd. Great parents, a wonderful woman who married me, a beautiful daughter— extremely lucky. You understand. Do I want it to all end? No. Will it end at some point?—of course. I'm not afraid though. I need you to know that. More importantly, I want you to know I'll be strong if I get the chance. I'll fight to get better; I can do this."

Dr. Anisee looked deeply at me, "I came down to talk one last time before making my decision. We can't take everyone—we can only take patients who are ready, who can make it through, who have a large life within. I'm putting you on the national donor list Monday."

I gave her a hug. "Thank you. I'll fight as hard as I can for you. I promise."

We sat quietly for a moment or two. She didn't get up to go; she sat for a bit longer. I asked her about stem cell research and if they were working with lung stem cells. She said, "We are closer than ever, but it's still far away. We hope it will come faster than we think; we just don't know."

"Want to know my dream goal?"

It was dark now, and the tops of the buildings were silhouettes. "Tell me."

"I want to get a double-lung transplant, have it go well, live ten more years, have them create stem cell lungs from my bone marrow like you said, come back to you, get new lungs, and live another ten years."

"That's a wonderful thought, Robert. I want to be here for that."

I smiled and knew she had to go. She had been with me for an hour.

"Thanks so much for all you've done for me and my family. I can't put it in words right now."

She stood up and gave me another hug. "Kristen will discharge you from here tomorrow and explain everything you need to know. I'll talk to you soon, as well. Keep working out. Get strong. Build up those legs!" She smiled and walked out the door with a small wave of one of her red gloves.

At Camp CYO in 1959 with my trusty mitt.

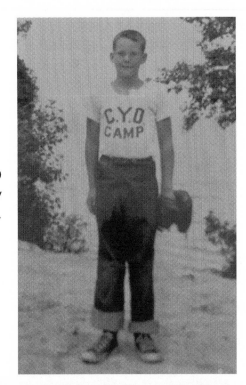

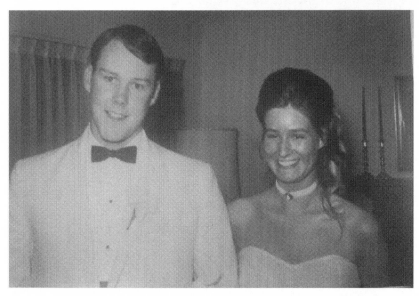

Jackie and I head for our senior prom in 1968.

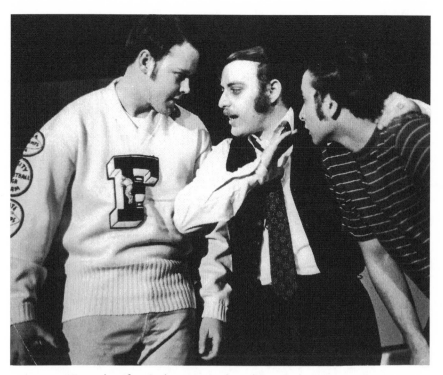

"Death of a Salesman" by the Michigan State
Theatre Department, 1970.

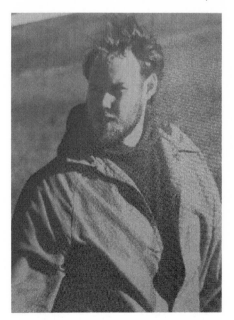

Coaching cross-
country in 1975.

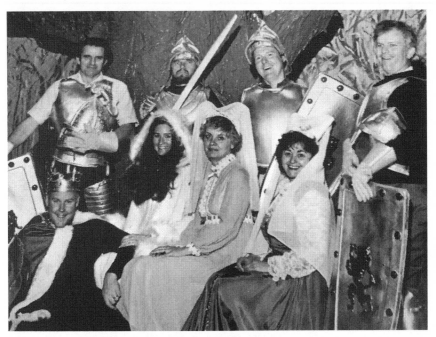

Director's snapshot of the "Camelot"
spring musical, 1985.

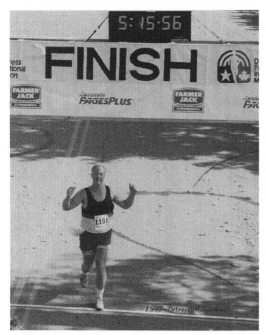

Finishing
the Detroit
Marathon,
1987.

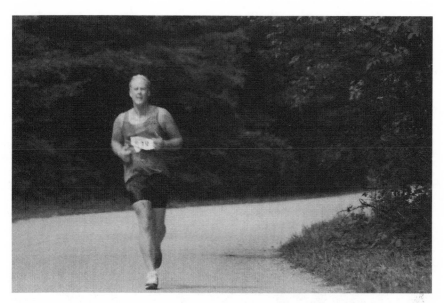

Running the Boyne Mountain Iron Man, 1988.

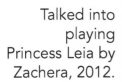

Talked into
playing
Princess Leia by
Zachera, 2012.

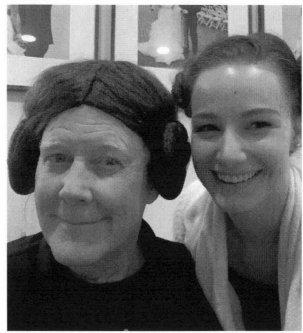

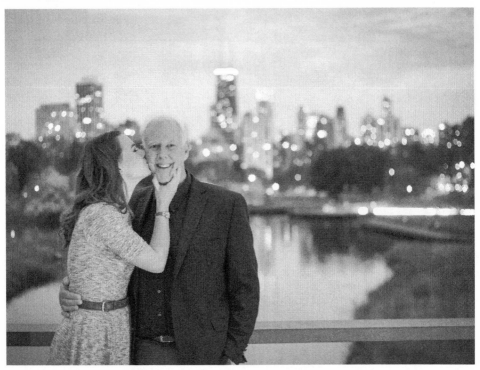

Giving dad a kiss in Chicago, 2015.

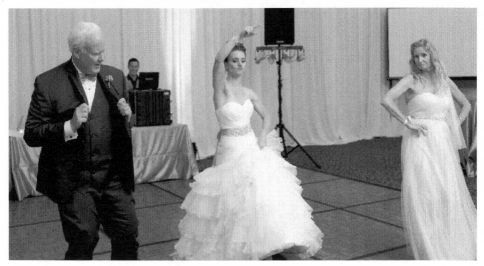

Dancing to Bruno Mars at Zachera and
Ryan's wedding, 2015.

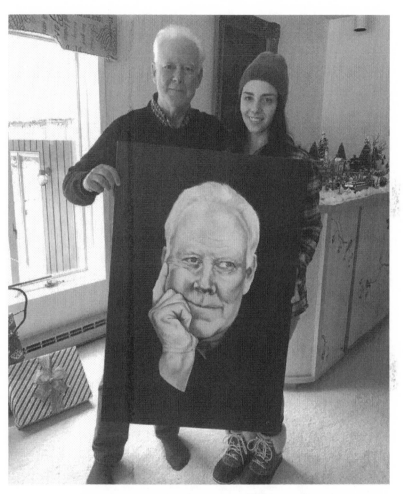

A portrait painting by one of my students,
Lanie McCarry, in 2016.

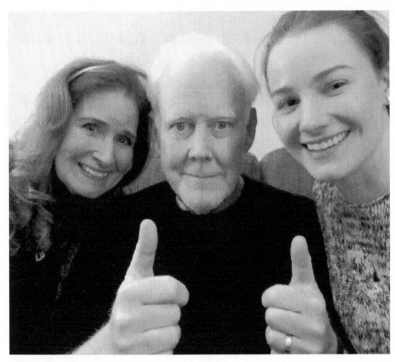

Thumbs up! First day out of the hospital, 2016.

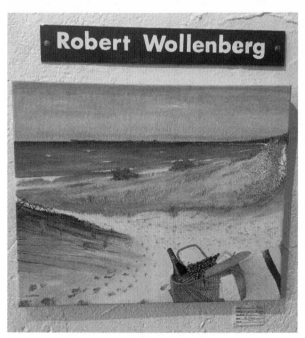

My first painting – "Picnic at Sturgeon Bay," 2017.

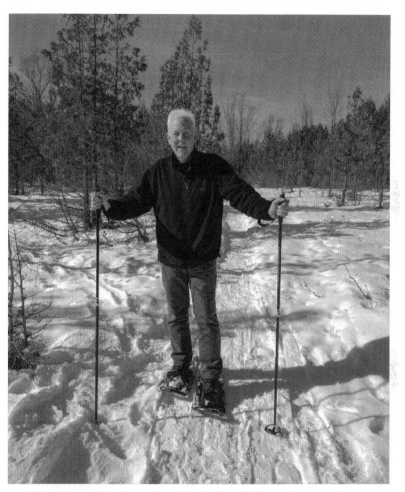

Snowshoeing the second year "out," 2017.

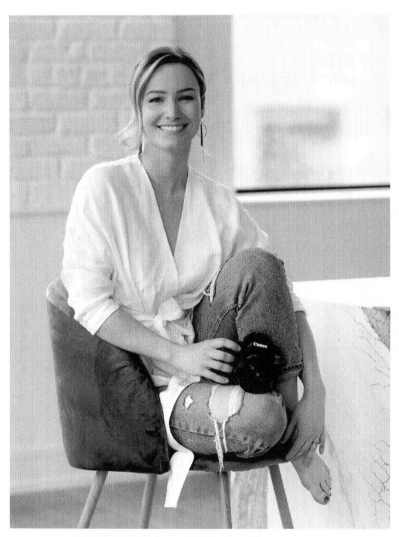

Zachera in her photo studio, 2018.

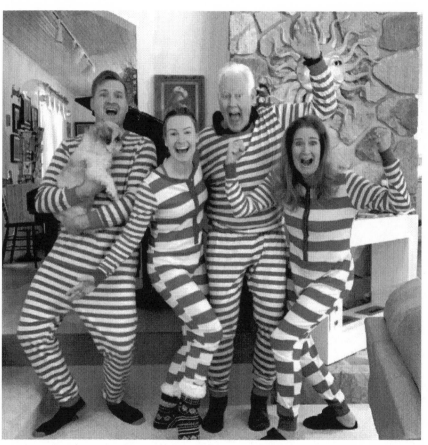

It was a crazy Christmas in 2019.

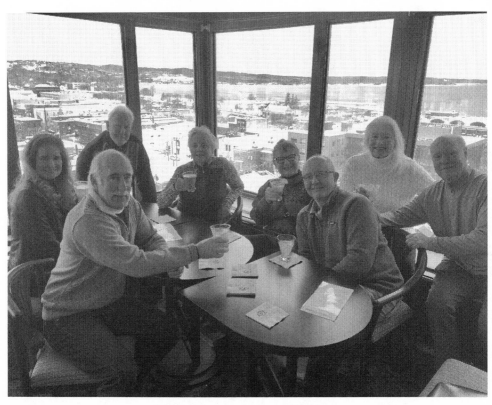

My support group, 2019.

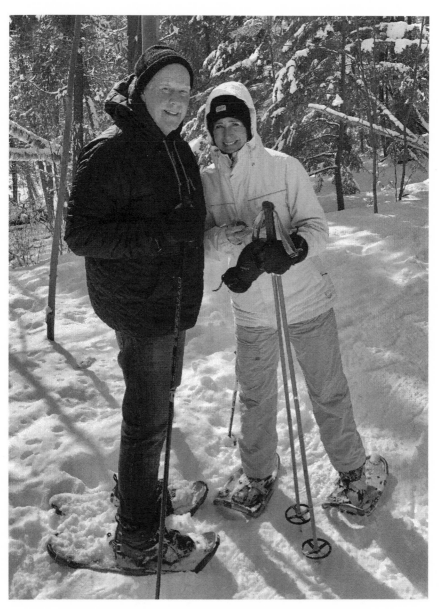

Snowshoeing the fourth year "out," 2020.

TWO
POST

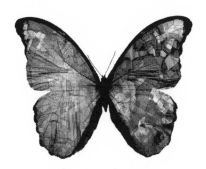 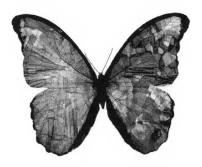

17

The Night Of...

He's quite a ways from walking outside. He wants to, but isn't up to it. He's staying on Tylenol and not going back to the strong meds. I think it's going to be so good for him. Drank something called Kionex or 120 ml of something that was to lower his potassium level. Thursdays, he takes extra Vitamin D and calcium. Wonder why only Thursdays? Clear sunshine—not overcast. He slept through five hours, which is better. Weighed himself...210 pounds, up three pounds from after surgery. He weighs himself nude so he'll weigh less. Ha! Talked to nurse about feeling bad and she said it was typical side effects after stopping Norco. William, his physical therapist, came to the room for first day. Glucose test was on target. Pain is under control, but he didn't feel good today. Said he felt like he didn't have any energy. Did crosswords and slept. He sleeps a lot. I talked to Mom and Dad for a long time on my phone and then did some painting. Tried to eat dinner at The Windsor instead of the hotel's free business dinners, which are pretty basic. It takes a lot to get Em down to the lobby where The Windsor is. It has a nice menu, lots of things he can have, but he didn't eat much. His appetite has gone up and down. He says things he used to like don't taste good. – Jac

The doctors said, "Whenever we are notified and have donor

lungs that fit your profile, you will receive a call from us immediately. When you get this call, do not eat anything, especially anything spicy. Get to the hospital as quickly as you can. Since you're on the donor list, you need to stay only fifteen to thirty minutes away from our hospital at all times."

After all the doctors, appointments, waiting, tests, waiting, more tests, and days of uncertainty…the time had come to receive a double-lung transplant.

All I know is, Ol' Mother Superior's assessment of my mental state as an eight-year-old student hauntingly showed up the night we received the call. For the record, Mother Superior was never right—my mother was right—but on this particular night my brain did slightly malfunction. To start with, I broke every rule the doctors gave me regarding arriving at the emergency door. To be fair, whilst enjoying our night out with two great friends who had driven down from up North to Chicago to visit us, we hadn't the faintest idea the call was forthcoming. No one knew it was "the night of…"

First of all, Ryan and Zachera wanted to take our friends Jim and Evelyn with us to this really bizarre ethnic restaurant not far from their condo in Ukrainian Village. Once there, we ordered all sorts of curious dishes, passing each concoction around so everyone could have a taste. I didn't recognize any of it. As a matter of fact, nothing even tasted or looked familiar whatsoever. This, of course, meant my dinner—and stomach—now contained foods spanning the globe—wild spices, weird gravies, items related to eyeballs, and bread that could be a cleaning sponge. Justttt what the surgeons wanted if I got the call!

To add to my gastronomical fray, after we left MomboNickiAdddaaaa or some weird name, we all headed down to a local gourmet ice-cream shop nearby with some woman's name like Ellen's or Linda's or something. They had ice cream in flavors like Corn and Cream, and Asparagus with Caramel—desserts that matched right up with our weird dinner.

Unfortunately, the ice cream shop was closed. It was now after ten p.m., so we figured we'd go back to our hotel and call it a night. But, after a few minutes of walking, Jim said, "Hey, you know there's a Cheesecake Factory right down the street from our hotel on Michigan Avenue. Let's Uber back and go there!"

Everyone agreed and off we went with stomachs sloshing a mighty strange mix of ingredients around. Arriving at the Factory, we shared enormous sundaes piled high with whipped cream, Sanders hot fudge sauce, nuts, berries, the whole nine yards. After our now second onslaught, we veritably rolled back to the hotel, said goodnight, and headed to our different rooms to prepare for a good night's sleep with, no doubt, strange dreams.

In our room, Jackie asked me about tomorrow's plans with our friends and proceeded to put her nightgown on, get ready for bed, and brush her teeth. I sat on the couch looking at the *Chicago Now* magazine every hotel in every city seems to have laying on their coffee table. I was so full, staying up awhile reading seemed an intelligent choice.

Since it was now around 11:30 p.m., the ring of my cellphone startled me. I thought it might be one of our friends wanting to plan something fun for tomorrow, but a different voice said, "Hello, is this Robert Emmet?" It didn't sound like a spam caller because whomever it was sounded close, clear, and there weren't people in the background talking in a different language. Bam! It hit me. 11:30 p.m. This could be it: the call.

"Ah...yes, it is," I said.

A voice said, "This is Cynthia, one of your nurses from MMHMM's lung transplant team."

Jackie yelled from the bathroom while brushing her teeth, "Wooooo...cal...n? ooos cal ssss tim a naaaa?"

I yelled back to her, "Wait! Wait a minute! I'm on the phone!!" and then said to Cyn...something, trying to stay calm, "Excuse me. You mean, you're calling from the hospital? This is the call?

"Yes it is, Robert. This is 'the call.' The real thing. We have donor lungs for you. We need you to arrive at MMHMMM's emergency entrance as soon as you can. I will be waiting for you there. Again, this is Cynthia."

Jackie yelled from the bathroom again. Cynthia continued her instructions, "Make sure to bring your pack of clothes and necessities—your Go Bag we talked about in clinic—and your lung team files and papers, okay? I know who you are and I'll be waiting for you right by the emergency room's revolving door."

Jackie came into the room with her toothbrush in her mouth. "Wooo uuuur tlkingg toooo?"

I was in a panic. A good panic, but a panic all the same. This was it! This was...good! I didn't know. I didn't know what to think. Was this good? It was what we were waiting for. The real thing. It was happening! This fast! It had only been eight days, and they told us it could take months and months. I was scared and excited all at the same time.

"We gotta go!!" I yelled in a high-pitched voice.

Jackie tried to talk through her toothpaste, "Whaaaa? Goooo eerrrrr?"

"We gotta go!" was all I could yell. I started to frantically look for the pre-packed, special edition, all everything Quick Go Bag they told us to put together. First, the closet in the bedroom! Jackie finished what she was doing and came into the room and found me kneeling down in the hotel closet, "Jac! Hey! There's a pile of dirty clothes in here. Is this where the Quick Go Bag is?!"

Jac grabbed my arm and said, now audibly, "Go where? What's going on? I'm not going out again no matter what our friends want! I just changed my clothes, my hair's a mess from all that wind, andddd, it's almost midnight!!"

"The call...the call!! We've got to go, we've got...to go!!"

Jackie said, "Calm down, what do you mean 'the call'? From who? The hospital?"

"Yessss!! The call!! We've got to go!! Come on, they want me at the emergency entrance right now!!"

Jackie shouted, "Oh my God! They want you now?! Which entrance?!"

We were both shouting! It was like we were having a baby! Same crazy!

"Hell if I know, we'll figure it out when we get over there! We gotta go!!"

"There's about three different emergency entrances! Which one?!"

I shouted, "Where's the Quick Go Bag??"

Jackie shouted, "The Quick Go Bag? That was your job! What did you do with it?"

"I don't know! It's got to be here somewhere! Maybe we left it in that other hotel room!?!" I yelled.

Jackie said, "Other hotel room? What? You mean when they switched us?? We brought everything from there. I checked! Was it a blue and grey gym bag?"

I let out a frustrated, "I know it's blue and grey cuz it's my bag!"

Jackie yelled, "No!! Ahhhh! Just tell me the colorrrr! @#! It's not in this closet. It might be...wait!....I think it's behind the couch!!" Jackie ran into the other room and started to pull the couch away from the wall.

"Really?! You put the Quick Go Bag where no one could find it?!" I shouted.

"I knew where it was!" Jackie retorted.

"Oh my God! What if you weren't here? Then what would I have done! @#!" I shouted from the closet.

"Ok, got the bag!! I thought you said we have to go!!" Jackie said.

I said, "We doooo!! But we need the Go Bag!!"

"Got it!@#!"

"Where did you put it?!" I screamed.

"For God's sake, I got it!! We have to go!!" Jackie yelled back.

"We need the papers!" I shouted. "They said bring the papers!"

"What papers?!" Jackie asked pulling out the not-so-quick Quick Go Bag from behind the couch.

I went mental. All I could do was stand there. "I don't know. The papers!! Shit!!"

Jackie yelled back, "We gotta go! We'll get the papers later."

"What if they need the papers!?"

"They won't! Jesussss!! We gotta go!" Grabbing the hotel key / card / plastic thing, out we went.

There were three elevator doors in our floor's hallway. Or course, we got the slow one and some juvenile pecker heads had pushed a bunch of floor buttons when they got off as a joke. We made it to the hotel lobby sometime the next day—or what felt like it. On the way down, Jackie called Zachera and let her know what was happening.

The hospital was right across the street, so we hurriedly entered through some revolving doors and ran up to the information desk. An older gentleman who was reading a book looked up, took his bookmark, and judiciously placed it on the page he was reading. He then said in a slow motion, molasses voice, "Cannnn I help... you?"

Jackie said excitedly, "We need the entrance to the emergency area."

The gentleman said, seeing we weren't hurt or passing out on the floor, "Mossss people...they...get there by ambulance...hehehe," His laugh was low and leisurely. "But...y'all can walk in...just as well...I suppppose...hehehe...Now, thaaaa'ssss funny..." Jackie was going to have a fit.

As always, she tried to be cordial, but intensely said, "Where is it??"

"Oh.... It's right over there. Wait, do you need your parking ticket stamped?"

We both shook our heads. "No, thanks."

"Alrighty then...you go.... right through over that-a-way...See... right through there...those double doors. Thaaaa's the emergency room entrance. You're practically there right now."

A sort of hiss/huff came out of Jackie's mouth at the same time. She had been stressed about the call, this moment, and it was going in super slow motion. We hustled towards the revolving doors. Cynthia was standing just inside, as she had instructed, and said, "Are you Robert? Robert Emmet?"

I said, "Yes!!"

Cynthia said, "And you're Jackie, yes?"

Jackie nodded and then Cynthia said, "We're going to head right down this way."

We followed Cynthia as she took us to the admitting area. Cynthia explained what was going to happen next in a much quicker cadence than the gentleman at the information counter, but nothing was sinking in. We were too stressed, excited, geeked, worried, and perplexed all at the same time.

A lady behind a Plexiglas window asked for my name and birthdate, banged on her copy machine, and then shoved about ten pieces of paper out through a slot. She said to bring them back when filled out. I rolled my eyes and Ms. Plexiglas kind of smirked. Cynthia, who had been talking to someone on her cell, stepped up and said, "This is Robert Emmet. He's all set. His information is all logged and ready. Please mark his admittance at 11:47 p.m. and I'll take him from here." Cynthia took my arm and guided us through the white hospital maze.

Jackie and I looked at each other like, "Wow, that was cool. MMHMMM must have their stuff together." They knew my name and everything. We took an elevator to the sixth floor and, after Cynthia stopped at the floor's main desk, a young man said he would take us down to our room. Earlier, after we ate our infamous dinner, Ryan had Ubered back to Boka, the restaurant where he worked, to finish up that day's financial reports. Zachera called Ryan as soon as she heard about the call and let him know I was being admitted. He left Boca immediately and headed back downtown.

To say prep work started on me right away would be an understatement. From the moment we entered our room on the surgery floor, I felt like John Glenn being placed in his capsule. Nurses were on autopilot: moving machines, setting up IVs, handing Jackie the infamous blue gown / puffy shower-cap set, and telling me to take all my clothes off, checking blipping screens, rotating dials, and turning on room monitors. No chit-chat.

I'm not sure why, but I was strangely composed. We had been yelling, rushing, and nervous, but now I was calm. This was it. What came over me was—I had signed up for this; it was my intent. This was it. *I'm goin' in.*

There was all this hustle and bustle, in-and-out going on around me...and then all of a sudden...the staff disappeared. I asked Jackie, "Did anybody say anything? What's the deal?"

Jackie said, "They just said to wait."

"Just wait? I thought we were headin' in?"

Zachera said, "That was prep, Dad. Surgery will give us the go-ahead when it's time."

Lying under warm blankets, I said, "Oh." and started playing with the up-and-down button of my hospital bed. I could go up and down pretty fast and it even slanted to one side or the other, which I decided not to play with because I might roll off.

Jackie said, "You're going to break that," so I stopped.

The pre-surgery room was ice cold and when Ryan arrived, Zachera and Jackie went in search of blankets. Ryan and I discussed his work and the Chicago Bears. At one point he asked, "What do you think? I mean, about all of this?"

"Ya know, it's ok. I want to do this. It's going to go ok. I've been a pain in the ass for you guys the last month or so, first staying at your place, and then having you guys drive downtown all the time."

"Not at all," Ryan said. "No problem whatsoever. Besides, you're always taking us to dinner all the time! We love that!"

We laughed, and Zachera and Jackie walked in with exactly one blanket. "It's all we could find. Has anyone come back yet?"

Ryan said, "Nope. Maybe somebody will bring some blankets. It's friggin' freezing in here!"

Time was going by and we all wondered why it was taking so long. Finally, a nurse walked in and said, "They are transporting your lungs right now. Two of our doctors examine the donor lungs presented and then send us an 'ok' in terms of whether or not they're a good fit for you. They believe it shouldn't be too long until we're ready." An image of an angel taking me down a soft, cloudy path slipped into my mind, then back out. This was not a thing of myths; this was as real as it gets.

Ryan immediately asked the nurse, "Is there any chance we could get some blankets? It's really cold in here."

The nurse said, "Sure, I'll get some sent down to you," and left. We all talked about something for a while; I can't remember. About twenty minutes later an orderly walked in with four blankets, saying, "Boy, you guys must be really cold."

I said, "Yeah, I'm warm as toast, but they're shivering."

The warm blankets put me to sleep, but I woke up once and saw Jackie, Zachera, and Ryan wrapped up in blankets like babies in an OB ward. Jackie was in a chair, Zachera was in an even smaller chair, and had propped up my suitcase to hold her legs. Ryan was curled up in his blanket on the floor looking extremely uncomfortable. I couldn't even see his face. Then I fell back to sleep.

Liftoff time finally came around six a.m. All of a sudden someone woke me up and said they were taking me down to surgery. Jackie jumped up as Zachera and Ryan were coming out of whatever little state of sleep they were in. Two staff orderlies said to Jackie, "Ok, say your goodbyes. We're taking him now." Just that fast.

It all happened at once. Jackie, Zachera, and Ryan followed me down this corridor to some automatic doors leading to the operating area. The orderlies hit the chrome remote button on the wall and two large doors swung open. Zachera held my hand with Ryan close behind. Jackie leaned down at the last second to give me a kiss, and, as they took me through the doors, I raised my fist up, letting my family know I was ready to do this, and disappeared down a dark hallway. I knew the odds, but was ready to throw Zachera's dream no-hitter.

Moving down the hallway, my gurney traveled through another set of automatic doors and entered this enormous room. I remember believing *I'm in the Kennedy Space Center!* probably because of the drugs going through the IV. It was a room the likes of which I've never seen—wires, tubes, TV screens, masked people, bags of liquid, people giving orders, people with weird tools, very bright lights, and cold, cold air. There were monitors everywhere, like a gigantic sports bar.

A vivid memory came into my mind as we wheeled into the actual operating room. I was a young boy watching John Glenn's capsule bobbing in the ocean after he returned from space. They kept calling Glenn's mission astonishing and remarkable. Walter Cronkite's deep and slow voice came from our little black-and-white Zenith TV: "And now, we see the courageous and brave astronaut John Glenn being lifted out of his small space capsule. He gives the world a wave of 'ok' and has a much-deserved smile on his face for his heroic flight and recovery."

Would they find me in the vast ocean? Would I have a recovery? Would I make it and wave the thumbs-up "ok"? Glen had headed into a cold and foreboding place and then came back. Would I do the same? People were talking, giving all sorts of orders, orders, and then…then…everything…every th…faded…fad…fa…f…to black.

When you think about it, a person going through a double-lung transplant or any major surgery is on a space journey. My wonderful daughter sent me David Bowie's "Space Oddity" to listen to weeks before my transplant. "Ground Control to Major Tom…" I played it over and over, not realizing how much it paralleled my experience.

I'm stepping through the door
And I'm floating in a most peculiar way…

Kristen, our PA, told Jackie, Zachera, and Ryan it would be a long 10 or 11 hours of surgery and suggested they go back to the hotel, get something to eat, and some rest. Once back, Zachera and Ryan immediately laid down and feel asleep. Jackie was too anxious and worried so she met our visiting friends for a pre-arranged breakfast downstairs. Jim and Evelyn were totally shocked to hear what had happened during the night. They were just packed up and ready for their drive back to Boyne City.

As the morning moved on, Ryan had to go back to work and

Zachera needed to go back to their condo to take their little dog, Oliver out. Jackie's mind was a whir. She couldn't just sit, so she went for a long walk outside on the sidewalks surrounding the hospital. That way she would be close.

Around noon, Jackie received a call from a surgery nurse who said the doctors had completed one lung and things were "going well". The nurse said she would call later that afternoon to let Jackie know when it was time to come back to the surgery floor and meet with the doctors. Jackie immediately called Ryan and Zachera with the positive news, "Got a call! The nurse said, the doctors think he's halfway home!" She didn't let thoughts of what the surgeons might tell them later even enter her mind. It was not time.

The call did come around 4:30 pm and Jackie, Zachera, and Ryan all met in the waiting room for the surgeons. They looked at each other – the outcome was going to change their lives and each one knew it. Their thoughts sat waiting… Jackie called her mom and dad to tell them what she knew…They waited…

Finally, all of a sudden the doors swung open and all four of the transplant team's doctors, plus Kristen and Paul, headed towards them…with, as Jackie described later, "smiles grinning from ear to ear!"

Like Glenn's flight into the unknown, ten surgery hours later my incredible doctors sent me hurtling back to Earth.

"I knew right away you were ok!" Jackie said, describing the look on my doctors' faces as they walked towards them. We were all aware of the consequences. It could go have gone either way—fifty-fifty—but they told Jackie, Zachera, and Ryan I had come through with flying colors; the surgery had gone exactly as planned. In fact, the surgeons said, "Robert's lungs are the best fit we've ever seen in years of transplant surgery. They lined up and fit perfectly!"

Because of brilliant surgeons and all the family support providing the love a person could ever wish for, I came back through those swinging doors—this time from the other side. There was a long way to go, but I was back…and alive.

18

Recovery

The doctors said he's doing well. His vitals are steady. He made it through. They were the words I had been waiting for since the beginning. They made me feel wonderful inside. He made it. I held my breath; my body tense all this time waiting…waiting…and now I can try to exhale. It's hard to write this in my journal because it's been so much. They let Zachera, Ryan, and I peek into his ICU room. We couldn't go in because they were too busy setting up all the machines that were keeping him alive. He was looking our way, but I don't think he could see us. It was like we were in a dream. Standing there in the hallway, I gave Zachera one of the longest hugs I've ever given her. It made me feel so wonderful inside to have Zachera and Ryan there with me. I couldn't imagine doing all of it alone. – Jac

For the record and for those of you who noticed the word "terrifying" in this book's title, this is probably the time to explain in very, very layman's terms what exactly took place during my double-lung transplant. So, here goes. Remember, this is only my understanding of what happened. Remember, where was I? In La La Land lying on my back with tubes goin' every damn which way and my eyes and mouth taped shut. Soooo, what do I know? Nothing. Therefore, this is what happened after the national anthem was played.

In a nutshell: the hospital got a call from the national organ donor association that a set of lungs had been donated by a family who had a family member die. Two surgeons from my hospital somehow went to where these donor lungs were located to check them out regarding the shape they were in, their size, and all sorts of other things I know nothing about. No telling where those two doctors were when they decided the donor lungs were, as they put it, "a good fit" (what they told Jackie) and brought the lungs back to my hospital in a Target cooler (fineeee—ok—probably wasn't from Target). Meanwhile, back at the ranch, the hospital staff got me all strapped in on the gurney and off we went through the famous swinging doors I told you about. Then, as I understand it, as the lungs in said Target cooler were being transported to my hospital, the staff prepped me, which is a staff term for what's done to a turkey on Thanksgiving morning. Needles in arm, dripping stuff in tubes, lots of celery salt, tons of anesthetics, tablespoons of pepper, doctors giving orders, nurses going in and out, everyone talking at once. Soon, I was ready with chest exposed (and probably everything else) and being lifted on the count of three onto a stainless-steel table. In rolls a cart with the two lungs on ice like shrimp cocktail, and all five surgeons got together to check'em out. They then murmured a collective "hummm," huddled up for a pep talk, clapped hands, and ran out onto the field.

Ok, brace yourself or go in the other room because this part is graphic. Don't read this if you can't ride rollercoasters, get nauseous, woozy, or the word "queasy" bothers you in any way.

Are you sure?…ok…

So, evidently, the doctors figured out how to keep me breathing or oxygen in my blood somehow, then mailed my blood somewhere to wait until needed, in a machine or something. (This is soooo incomplete and wrong, but it's all I've got for you.) Then they did something with my heart, put it in a jar, or a nice snug, warm place and commenced cutting my chest open from armpit to armpit. It's called a "clamshell incision" because that's what it looks like, I guess. So, once that was finished, they opened up everything and took a look-see. They had to cut my sternum, which holds all your ribs together, in half so they could lay open each side of my rib cage wide enough to get the lungs—the largest organs in the human body—in and out. Some frigging way, they took one bad lung out, put it in a bucket or whatever, and attached one of my new donor lungs. Remember, this is no minor organ—this is an organ that takes in everyday air, separates the oxygen from all this other stuff, then sends the other stuff out into the world so trees and plants can eat it. So, while my blood was on holiday and my heart was in rehab, they checked whether my first new lung was hooked up ok. That was the first five hours.

Then, they got into the Target cooler, had a snack, maybe some Cheetos, and something to drink. Preferably non-alcoholic.

The next five hours, they saw how the ol' first lung was doing and then repeated. Pretty soon both lungs were hooked up, tubes, gas gauges, airways, oil pans, and such were checked and re-checked. A couple of nurses helped the surgeons pull my rib cage back together, bound up my sternum with some kind of dis-solving string, and...zing-zang-zoom...they stitched up my old, weird lookin' chest! Back to ICU I went!

That's what surgeons do while you're out buying groceries and chatting with the bakery lady...Just like that...Bam!

Incredible. No words.

Surgeons headed home, stopped at a local brewery for a beer or three. No beer for me, just the long road back to consciousness. Wow.

Wow and wow.

After my double-lung transplant, the first time I was aware of anything was in the ICU recovery room—that strong and vital word again, recovery. Floating back into existence from a place far away; it was foggy. Lots of fog wherever it was. Wasn't outside. There was movement around me. In time, there was: a room, people talking—sounds, not right there, but near me. Not sure whether a wizard stuck his head in the open window, but I remember moving my eyes to the right and left and they were all there, just like in the movie. I tried to figure out where I was and what I was doing on my back in a strange bed? What happened next was exhilarating—I fell back asleep.

So, it was the fall back-to-sleep /wake up / fall back-to-sleep train. This was followed by the looking from side to side, thinking 'hmmm,' and falling asleep again train to Albany. What's really weird is, I distinctly remember doing the wake up / sleep thing and vaguely wondering when things would begin to move forward. It was like, "Is this all I do? Fade in...fade out...fade in...Shouldn't I be doing something like lifting weights or playing a board game? I'm just lying here."

As it turns out, what was really happening was the hospital staff was giving me big-time drugs so I wouldn't wake up in the middle of the night and yell "WTF!!" at 400 decibels! Hospital staff know stuff like that. They know when you need to be totally incoherent and on top of some weird mountain.

There was a lot going on around me by design, but none of it was registering...that I knew of. Each time I woke up, there was less fog, and a little bit more focus. I started to make out different people, and finally those people were Jackie, Zachera, and Ryan looking in my room from the hallway door. It seemed like it was the first real thing I understood. I wanted to motion to them to "come in!" but couldn't move, couldn't say anything. I had "nothin'," as the saying goes.

That image, the image of them in the doorway, will be forever etched in my mind. The three most important people in my life... just peekin'. Peekin' in like I was a special exhibit at the zoo and they were just trying to get a glimpse through the crowd. Like they might ask for my autograph. Seeing them was one of the most exhilarating moments of my life because I knew somehow, somewhere inside...if I was truly seeing them...I had made it back.

Eventually, accepting my location and that nurses and doctors were working with me made sense. I was only mentally taking in 20 percent of the show. It was like looking through small old opera glasses from the worst seat in the theatre and trying to understand the musical *Hamilton*.

The next day, Jackie and Zachera walked in my room and up to the bottom of my Tilt-o-Matic hospital bed. Jackie moved closer and put her hand on my arm. It was the touch I was waiting for. I was on the other side of those large swinging surgery doors—the doors that swallowed me, the doors I fought to let me back out. I was alive and Jackie and Zachera and Ryan were there. It was Dorothy at the end of *The Wizard of Oz*, "and you and you and you were there. All of you!"

Jackie told me later, laughing, they weren't in my room more than a minute before I asked for help. She said I kept trying to move my hand sort of towards me. Jackie asked over and over, "What do you need? What do you want?" but I couldn't talk. I kept making the same hand motion. It was like playing charades when your team can't guess the answer. Jackie came up close to my ear, "Are you hot?" I moved my hand up and down. She knew me. After asking the nurse if it was okay, Jackie and Zachera pulled down the multitude of blankets covering my now sweaty neck and Jackie said I became less agitated.

Jackie came to my room every day. Ryan had to work and so did Zachera, but they came when they could, which always put a smile on my face. There were medical maneuvers, tests, gurneys, elevators, connect the dots, wires, more tubes, lots of nurses/doctors, people looking at me from every conceivable angle. Lots of bests and worsts. (I don't think "worsts" is the plural form, but just let it go—like whether or not to eat sausage.)

Soon things were becoming more coherent. There were all sorts of things the staff wanted me to do. Lots of gadgets to either breathe into, sit on, or play with whilst they watched. Some with little balls going up and down in a tube. Hospitals must have miles of tubes. There were tests and more tests, one right after another. Drawing what time it was on a clock, raising my right arm, pointing to my catheter. (No, they didn't ask me to do that, but I damn well knew where it was.) Fun stuff. Then I'd sleep some more.

Not much to write about during this time of my recovery because, as I've said, they kept me foggy on purpose. Some things stood out: sitting up for the first time, putting my feet on the floor, taking a step or two, my first transcontinental trip to the bathroom, and shuffling the halls, leaning on my metal walker thing with buckets and monitors hanging from it.

The rest: fogggg.

19

Zachera's Dream

So lucky to be here in this nice hotel instead of the hospital. It's right across the street from MMHMMM, so I feel so much better being closer to Em. How cool is that! Can't imagine being farther away. I can walk to his room in minutes! Sort of like a home away from home...well, not, but...Room has a view of the city, a coffee pot that actually holds more than two cups, and because it's a hotel, they will clean the room whenever I ask. Sometimes Zachera comes downtown and stays the night with me.—Jac

One lesson in life I've learned is, "The more we know, the more we know we don't know." I used to discuss this saying with my students. We learn something and think we've really got it, but what we really learn is our new knowledge opens up a vast realm of knowledge we don't know.

Walking across MSU's campus, I'd gaze at all the buildings of knowledge, all the different learned areas. I'd think, *How wild is it that I could spend my complete life learning everything in that one building over there and when I finished, that building would still have ten times more to learn. And, that's just one building. There are hundreds of buildings like that on campus. There's so much to know, so much more we don't know.*

Because of this, never discount any new thought or idea. We

have no idea what there is to know…right now…this minute…let alone in the future. Never scoff at an idea someone talks to you about, because whether we think it could happen or not, we will never know…for sure.

When we were told about my prognosis and impending surgery, my daughter was extremely distraught. She was sure she was going to lose me because of the odds of living through a ten-hour, double-lung transplant. Since she was an only child, we have been extremely close and love each other very much. Talking to her about the reality of the situation and that we're all going to die someday did no good. Not even a dent. Zachera would have to come to her own base about my circumstance. I was proud of her because, at some point in her own way, she did.

Then one evening soon after my transplant, Zachera and I sat quietly in our small hotel room across the street from MMHMMM. Jackie was sleeping. It had been a long day after being at the hospital at 6:15 a.m. for my blood draw and blood clot scan. Zachera was tired and she had a photo shoot early the next morning when the light was good on the shores of Lake Michigan.

Regardless, she stayed up and we talked about my recovery and what a wild ride it had been the last few weeks. Her legs were curled up beneath her on the couch and we weren't getting into any sort of a deep conversation, just how the day had gone, what the doctors said, and what her upcoming photo shoot entailed.

After a lull, Zachera looked up and asked me to listen to something she had on her mind. If she had something on her mind, it meant she had been ruminating on it for days. She was like her mother; once latched onto something, it was going to be dealt with. I said, "Of course."

Zachera said, "Dad, I told you something happened to me in the early morning of your surgery, right. I woke up while they were operating. Obviously, I couldn't see you, but I knew you were lying on a hospital bed full of tubes, masks, and breathing machines. I jerked awake in my bed and sat right up. I had been somewhere."

I said, "What do you mean?"

"I had really been somewhere, to a place. People talk about dreams being thoughts just rolling around in your head and all, but this wasn't like that. I didn't want to tell you or anyone because everyone always makes fun of people who claim they 'see things' or...I don't know...had a strange dream they thought was real. But I had been somewhere."

"How do you know? What made you feel like that?" I asked.

"I was there."

"Where?"

"That's what I'm telling you, it was as real as sitting here right now. I was walking through one of the tunnels leading onto the field at Comerica Park; you know, where the Tigers play in Detroit. It wasn't like the stadium where you played—old Tiger Stadium—it was much newer. I didn't know where I was at first, but because you took me to Tiger games before, it slowly started to look familiar.

It was night time, pretty dark in the stadium, but there was one bank of lights shining on the infield. I could see the edge of the big, expansive outfield. It was so green and they had cut it so it looked checkered. It was shadowy and darker farther out. You could tell the stands were there, just couldn't make them out. It was scary, mostly because I had no idea how I got there.

Most of the light fell on the middle of the infield. I was out past first base and heard a sound coming from near the pitcher's mound. Someone was throwing a ball into some sort of net at home plate. A basket full of baseballs was on a stand next to a person grabbing one, winding up in a delivery, and throwing it quite fast into the large white net. The net already had ten or fifteen baseballs in it."

"What happened then?" I asked.

"I walked up towards the pitcher's mound and this young man turned and said, 'Hi.' It was you...I mean...that's the thing. You said, 'Hi, Bud,' like you always do, so I knew it was you. But...you were only about nineteen, the age you said you were when being scouted by the Tigers. You were thinner, had dark hair, but the same broad shoulders. You wanted to know if everything was ok. I didn't know what you meant. You smacked the ball into your glove a couple of times, wound up, and threw it really fast towards the net. It hit the metal holding up the side of the net with a large clang that echoed in the empty stadium. You took another ball from the pile and looked at me—looked right through me, it seemed."

Listening intently, I said, "What then?"

"As you looked at me, you said, 'Tomorrow, I'm going to throw a no hitter.' You were not boasting; it was calmer, like you knew for sure it was going to happen."

"And?" I asked.

Zachera said, "I know you think this wasn't real."

"No, go on."

"You threw another pitch, and…that's it. I woke up."

I said, "Nothing else happened?"

"Nope," Zachera said matter-of-factly.

"Pretty wild…a dream like that," I offered.

Zachera said adamantly, "That's just it, Dad. It wasn't a dream. It was real. It was a real moment. We were both there. You looked exactly like the picture you gave me when you played at Tiger Stadium when you were eighteen years old. I sat up in bed. I didn't know what to do, just waited there in my bed to figure it out. It didn't make sense, but it did. You knew you were going to get through your surgery, that you were going to be ok…and you let me know. You didn't want me to worry, so you found me—or I found you—in another time, another space. I swear that's what happened and I know exactly why. You've spent your whole life teaching me, protecting me, guiding and loving me. You knew I was in a bad place worrying about you dying, dealing with the possibility, thinking about what it was going to be like without you. Just Mom and me…alone. While you were unconscious, you found me—somehow, somewhere—to let me know you were going to make it."

We sat for a minute. I said, "Zachera, I don't know…I don't know"

Zachera answered, "I do…I was there."

20

The Thrilla in Manila

Heading to a blood-draw appointment tomorrow morning. Instructions: take Prograf at eight p.m., no food or drink after midnight. No meds in morning until after appointment. He tried another suppository this morning to get 'going' down there, but nothing. He's walking in the hallway some, but when two nurses came into our room, he conned them into taking an exercise bike out of the workout area and putting it next to his bed. Not sure if he'll be able to get up on it yet, but if he's talking people into doing stuff, I know he's getting better! The nurses could have gotten in trouble once the workout attendant found a bike was missing! No one ever said anything, though. I got to use it, too! I try to go for an hour, watching Ellen. So far I'm afraid to go running outside in the downtown parks because I don't want to be away from him that long. After taking morning meds, he took his Norco, nausea pills, and took his own shower for the first time without me in with him holding him up. I sat on the toilet seat next to the shower just in case he needed me or fell. It was scary. He's not supposed to let the shower spray hit his stitches directly. I just read my book. He was in there for what seemed like about two hours and looked like a prune when he got out, but who cares! He's doing it!! – Jac

The truth is, there are stories…people stories…but many are

never told. Some are libraries that no longer exist, a pile of burned wood. Here's a story Jackie mentioned in her journal excerpts. It was an emergency episode Jackie, Zachera, and I went through. Would this be an episode worth writing about? It was human, real, and turned out to be one of the funniest moments of my whole ordeal. It exemplified why I wanted to write—because stories count, people count. We all have human experiences—some sad, some happy, some funny, some downright weird and embarrassing. But they're all stories worth telling because—we were here. We experienced a million moments; we lived life.

So, this particular handy little moment in time ended up famous—not hospital famous like my nose-wire pulling incident now in the anals (spelled deliberately) of MMHMMM history, but famous at least within our family. It might also be indelibly etched in the mind of a couple young female nursing assistants who took part, as you'll see. No matter how each person involved in this incident felt or thought, for the record, this is an exact account of the event!

Somewhere around the seventh or eighth day after my double-lung transplant, I was discharged from the hospital and Jackie and I were holed up in the Homewood Suites Hotel approximately two hundred feet from MMHMMM. Luck. This hotel ended up playing a pivotal role in my recovery for the following reasons:

One: I was discharged from the hospital early solely because we were going to be—literally—next door to MMHMMM. Two hundred fifty feet at most.

Two: I wasn't in a hospital—major, major plus.

Three: Our northern Michigan home was a six-hour drive away, so Jackie could get home some, and it was close enough for friends to visit.

Four: Where else could I go? Homewood Suites became our home away from home for three months.

Five: Visiting the hospital two or three times a day for blood draws, checkups, procedures, x-rays, urine samples, more checkups, shots, pills, etc. took, miraculously, all of five minutes travel time—door to door—if that. Remember, we're talking downtown

Chicago. Traveling multiple times a day to and from the hospital in my condition from any farther distance would have been impossible. Don't even mention gridlock traffic, five million pedestrians, or parking. OMG.

Six: Homewood Suites served a complimentary business-dinner buffet weekdays from five p.m. to seven p.m. I couldn't go out for dinner to a restaurant—quite far from that—so when Jackie couldn't cook a Crock Pot meal in our hotel room, she walked downstairs and carried up two plates from the buffet.

Ok, some of these things might seem inconsequential, but they were much more important than they sound.

For quite a few days Jackie documented in her journal the fact that I wasn't eating much and wasn't going to the bathroom, a.k.a. sending the log to the saw mill, taking one, shitting, squatting, dropping a load, heading to the shitter, making sausage, etc. In the hospital, a nurse's approach to being constipated (not the nurse, the patient) usually goes like this.

"Hi, I'm your floor nurse for today. Pull my finger. Justtt kidding!! Name's Surguna. Chart's got 'no bowel movements.' Eat yo' prunes?"

"Yes, I did…I mean…eat the prunes…but…ah…nothing happened. Didn't go," I offered.

"Well, let's see if this here baby git those bowels a-going, um hmm," Surguna said, as she unwrapped a suppository the size of a large Tootsie Roll.

"Y'all turn ova; we put this torpedo where it need be goin'."

Rule 47—When you think your day is going well, it can change.

My internal constitution was in deep turmoil because of my situation—a.k.a. lung transplant, pills, pain, hospital food, guests, needles, tubes, walkers, procedures, bad TV, and the Detroit Lions. I spent what seemed like minutes, hours, days trying to, as we say in layman's terms, "go." The hospital calls it lots of things and really makes it sound serious when they put it on a form—"Patient experiencing extremely high level 87 percent colon blockage due to unilateral lack of H2O and fiber particles entering esophagus via ventral opening with anal sphincter under construction." What?

My system was closed for the holidays. Suffice to say, things weren't working out. Double negatives were fun at this juncture: "nothin' was goin' nowhere." Food was going in, but there was no out. Blocked like Governor Chris Christie's New Jersey Bridge. No doubt this gridlock was due, as I said, to the ghoulish combination of thirty-five pills a day (no exaggeration), lots of peanuts, cheese, anchovies, Underwood devil's ham, frozen soup, licorice, rubbery clams, and today's hospital Lunch Special!! Plenty o' fun to keep all twenty-two feet of colon busy and any living organism tangled in a FUBAR backup. (Google this old military acronym. They tell you the "F" stands for "fouled," but it doesn't.)

One day, when I asked a nurse about the pills-to-constipation ratio, she said very matter-of-factly, "Yep, that'll happen," which elicited a blank stare from me, like one of those stupid cellphone emojis.

"Easy for you to say in your bluey gown and puffy shower cap, with normal bowel movements!" I said in a snarky way. I was going to write, "snarkily," but I'm quite sure "snarkily" isn't a word. I kind of like it though. People know what you mean when you say "snarkily." That should count for something.

Alright, I didn't say the "Easy for you to say...," but wanted to. Come to think of it, there were a lot of snarky, below-the-belt comments I wanted to make when I was in this special intestinal situation. But, as a teacher during parent/teacher conferences quickly learns, you have to mince words when Mrs. Mackerel's little Johnny is a flaming asshole.

Getting back to the matter at hand, things in the nether region weren't working—the freeway was at a serious standstill—the drain was plugged—tickets to Fenway Park were not available (which makes no sense at all). After the fourth day of "packin' it in," a discussion ensued with my lung transplant team. They decided to make a move. "We need to x-ray his gastros. Call service for a gurney and get him down there."

Hmmm, I thought sarcastically, *Yeah, an X-ray will make me take a dump, for sureeee.* Another gurney ride was underway and I was down to X-ray in just a couple of hours. It was the x-ray room of all x-ray rooms—miles long, screens everywhere, leaded vests, people with gas masks and pink cones on their head—remember, I was on pretty strong narcotics. The Cone Head People suited up in their safe lead vests and left me, as usual, naked, blowing in the wind. Probably ok, right? This, of course, was now the twentieth time under the radiation blaster...is there a limit? After twenty times, does your urine glow?

After my uranium shot, there was a bit of a wait for the Uber gurney driver, followed by an interesting ride back/discussion about what it was like to live in Morocco. When we arrived back to Dr. Anisee's office, an x-ray of my twenty-two-foot colon was on full display illuminated by one of those backlit, white plastic panel jobs mounted on the wall. This was set up for the whole transplant team to view, including any waiting-room patients and people in line at Sam's Fine Donuts. The picture of my fudge-packed colon was right up there front and center and everyone, including the cleaning lady who was sneaking a quick look from the bathroom, was checking it out. I asked quietly so the guys in the donut line couldn't hear, "Constipation or...?"

Looking closely at the x-ray, Dr. Anisee turned her head slightly sideways, all the onlookers leaned in, took a deep breath, and waited..."Yep, you're pretty blocked up!" A big gasp came from the audience. For God's sake, this wasn't the final verdict of the OJ Simpson trial! #!

My condition wasn't caused solely from eating a lot of cheese the night before—you know, the Gino's pizza/sausage/wire incident. It was what every TV evening news ad break runs around dinner time. You know, it's either osteoarthritis problems or ads where a curiously familiar-sized and shaped "thing not to be named" is now a blue log moving left to right across your sixty-inch screen like a Disney ride. Making it blue doesn't disguise what it is supposed to be. Sorry.

After conferring with others in the room, and the cleanup lady just to make her feel needed, Dr. Anisee said, "Let's give you one more day to let things perk in there and then, if nothing happens, we'll decide what to do." This, of course, was code for, "If Mount Vesuvius doesn't erupt, evasive action must commence." I looked at Dr. Anisee and said, "Is this normal? Is this going to cause trouble?"

Dr. Anisee said, in her soft, sympathetic tone, "You're ok. Gotta run. We'll talk tomorrow." Dr. Anisee could have told me they were flying in five specialists and I wouldn't have worried. If she told me I was ok...I was ok. She was the best of the best.

Ok or not, my afternoon was uncomfortable. Wrestling, skiing, or tennis might have loosened things up, but none of that was happening in my present condition. Zachera came over that evening to help. I tried to eat what Jackie made for dinner in our hotel room's Crock Pot (there was no stove) but to no avail. Everything seemed to stop at the back of my throat. Swallowing was getting more difficult because my stomach was, at this point, a giant neon sign flashing "no vacancy." Problems were piling up.

By around ten p.m., I told Jackie and Zachera something had to be done or I was literally going to blow up. There was no waiting until tomorrow. Because I was now in a world of hurt, Jackie called the eighteenth-floor pulmonary department where Kristen worked, but because it was so late, everyone had gone home. Kristen always told us to call their lung transplant team's emergency number if anything went wrong...and it was definitely going wrong. I wore the number stamped in metal on my emergency wrist bracelet.

The call was answered by a nurse who said Dr. Anisee was in the hospital but was involved in surgery. Dr. Anisee would get in touch with her when she became available, and I should go to MMHM-MM's emergency room in the meantime.

This was the worst place in the world for a new lung transplant patient with an immune system of zero. It was like taking your dog to a flea festival. Trust me, it's not something for the faint of heart. Avoid at all costs. I'm not kidding.

First, we had to find the normal entrance to the emergency room, not the area where ambulances came speeding in with sirens blaring. We figured it out and checked in at the front desk situated in a large hallway with high ceilings that echoed. We were then guided to the actual entrance door.

This was around six days out from my transplant surgery and my body was extremely susceptible to the pick-your-flavor germ, disease, sick people stuff. My iffy situation called for sterile white sheets, spotless floors, polished bedpans, and gallons of Purell hand sanitizer, not big city emergency room. My purposely suppressed immune system was keeping my body from rejecting my new donor lungs. It was also suppressing my body's ability to ward off Rice Krispies, let alone killer germs. Think about it, emergency rooms are packed with very sick, unhealthy, bleeding, throwing up, sneezing, disease spreading, pissed-off people. This was *No Country for Old Men—With Transplants*...tenfold.

The hospital staff immediately set me in a wheelchair—like they do. Zachera, who was already in a highly stressed state knowing what we were heading into, pushed me down this long hall, with Jackie, as always, by my side. As we turned a corner and pushed through metal-sided swinging doors, we faced a huge room with close to one hundred people sitting in waiting chairs, standing slumped over, leaning on walls—sicker than shit. The type of sick is hard to explain. It ran the gamut. People were moaning, holding up arms, legs were bent over sideways and upside down. One family of three was crying—all of them. Old guys were leaning back with their eyes rolling, people were sobbing, one guy was moving around with his arms out, making the sound of an airplane. Orderlies were moving up and down the aisles trying to get to a guy who said he had a knife in his ear. If Dante was alive, he would have used this chaotic scene in his book, *Inferno*.

What was really bad, specifically for me, was every other person was coughing. The flu was in high season in Chicago and its nasty head was leering from every corner. Getting the flu, or much worse, pneumonia, in my condition flat-out couldn't happen. It couldn't even be on my radar—in any shape or form. As vulnerable as my body was, getting something serious on top of it could kill me. People say, offhandedly, "Oh, this or that might kill ya." My situation was not offhanded—it was straight-out fact.

As soon as we entered, Zachera said, "Oh my God, Dad, we've got to get you out of here. You can't be in here. You're going to get sick here." She told Jackie to wheel me behind her as she maneuvered her way up to the emergency desk at the other end of the enormous room. Jackie jockeyed my wheelchair as best she could through rows and rows of sick patients. As she tried to make her way, she banged the side of a man's chair and he screamed. I couldn't do anything to help. One old lady grabbed my arm, asking me to help her, and then she coughed towards me—a horrible, deep hacking cough. Others looked at us like, "Hey, where you going? I'm next. I was first!"

The aisle became too narrow for the wheelchair. The only thing Jackie could do to get me away from everyone was to quickly park me in some sort of niche by a side hallway. Our lung team had emphatically told us, "Whatever you do, don't let Bob get near anyone who is sick. He has a very, very low immune system—if he gets sick, his body won't be able to fight it." We were in the worst possible area we could possibly be.

Jackie stayed close and tried to get Zachera's attention so she'd know where we were hidden in the small alcove. She couldn't get Zachera to notice. From what Jackie could see Zachera was really angry and upset.

Somehow Zachera had fought to the front of the line. People were yelling at her, but she had to get me out of there. In a panicked voice, Zachera screamed to the nurse at the desk over the loud din, "My dad's had a double-lung transplant. He can't be here! Someone has to help me get him out of here!"

"Excuse me, but there are people in line," the nurse yelled back. The room was loud, and people were screaming.

"I don't care! My dad could die from being in here! He's had a double-lung transplant!"

"Miss, I can only do what I can here. What's his full name?"

Zachera came unglued. "Listen to me! STOP what you're doing and get Dr. Anisee on the phone! Get my dad in a room away from here!"

"Dr...who?"

"Dr. Anisee—ANISEE—She's his lung surgeon. She's head of his lung transplant team. I know she's here in the hospital tonight!"

"I'm sorry, but you have to fill out these forms before I can do anything," the nurse said.

"You can't call her? This hospital has no way of finding a doctor in an emergency situation?!"

"Excuse me, miss, but you'll have to fill out..."

That was it. Zachera knew she was getting nowhere, so she quickly switched gears. Running around behind the admitting desk, while the clerk's mouth dropped, Zachera grabbed someone in a white coat coming by. Maybe she might be a doctor or nurse who could help. "Excuse me!" Zachera said as she grabbed her by the arm. "My dad is in the middle of that." She pointed to the emergency room. "He just got a double-lung transplant, has no immune system. He can't be in there! Can you help me ??!!"

Zachera's move paid off. The woman in the white coat turned out to be one of the emergency doctors. She understood right away what Zachera meant about my suppressed immune system and lung transplant.

"Where's your father?" the doctor quickly asked.

"He's..." Zachera looked back, but we were gone. "He's right... down..." Her heart sank. We were nowhere to be seen. But then, off to the right, she saw Jackie's small hand frantically waving from a side opening halfway down the room. "There!! There's my mom! I'll go get him!"

The doctor stopped her and said, "No! Wait! See those doors there by where your dad is? Go back down there and wait for me. Trust me, I'll open the doors where he is and take him in—just give me one minute. We'll get him to a separate room. Go!"

Zachera moved through the packed aisles as fast as she could and found us. Just as she started to explain what was happening, the small side door opened and the doctor she had spoken to let us in. There were people yelling. The doctor shut the door quickly and opened a door to an empty room close by with a key fob.

"You guys stay here and I'll get back to you as soon as I can. It might take a while, but I won't leave you here. If someone asks why you're in this room, tell them it was Dr. Kennan's orders! His doctor is Dr. Anisee, right? I know who she is and I'll get word to her. We'll make sure your dad gets where he needs to go. Don't worry," she said, and left as swiftly as she arrived.

So, there we sat...trying to calm down. Zachera had taken care of me. Jackie and Zachera always took care of me. There's a reason why, when you're first interviewed as a possible transplant patient, they ask you all sorts of questions about your support group. This was an example of how you can't fully explain the importance of support. I truly believe I wouldn't have made it without Jackie and Zachera, Ryan, and all our friends who were the nucleus of my strong network.

Finally, someone knocked, poked her head in, and asked, "Are you a patient of Dr. Anisee's?"

"Yes!" Jackie answered immediately.

"Dr. Anisee wants me to take you to the next floor for your procedure. She wanted to apologized for your wait. She was in surgery."

Ever gracious, Jackie said, "That's certainly understandable. Thanks so much."

The nurse ushered us off to a much calmer place. No one was yelling. She gave directions to change into—you guessed it—one of those blue gowns, and to get up on the wax-papered table/bench/slab thingy. She said it might take a bit, but someone would come by to take care of the bowel procedure. They kept calling it "my procedure." I was going to get the first enema of my life. What a milestone! But how was thissss going to go? I quickly found out. Well, not so quickly, more like an hour later, but at least I was safe.

The emergency room ordeal had been traumatic and scary, but this problem, this whole rear-ender wasn't going to be fun. What it wassss going to be was embarrassing, no two ways about it. Of course it would be. Think about it—an enema: nurses, Jackie and Zachera, orderlies of some kind, and my naked ass sticking out like Roosevelt's face on Mount Rushmore.

Jackie and Zachera sat on two chairs in the room and I was on the patient table where the nurse told me to plop myself. She probably didn't use the word "plop," especially under the circumstances, but everything was revolving around the same theme. The first nurse didn't say much and left quickly, probably because she knew what was about to happen.

I sat quietly for a second or three and then turned to Jackie and Zachera, "You know, you can maybe...ah...go outside or for a walk when the nurse comes. From what they've told me, this isn't going to be pretty. You don't have to stay. I'll take it from here."

Jackie laughed, "You mean you don't want your wife and daughter present when you get this done?!"

"No—I—don't," I said, laughing along with the two of them. Laughing made me feel better. Actually, in truth, laughing jarred every one of my 8,977 stitches, and putting pressure on six days of not going to the bathroom was making me feel like the Hindenburg right before it exploded.

A very, very young nurse's aide finally came around the corner with a couple of sheets of paper in her hand. She couldn't have been older than, maybe, seventeen. Behind her stood her assistant, who was even younger, I'm guessing maybe three years old. They both had long straight hair, with teenage twinkles in their eyes. The leader of the two, who did all the talking, had a pink bow in her hair. She said, "Hi, I'm Jen," and then something about an enema. "Are you Mr. Robert Emmet?"

"Yes," I said, and answered the next question ahead of time. "April 6th, 1950."

"That's what I have! Cool!" Jen said in a perky voice. She was all excited that she had the right name. Did she know what she was being asked to do?

I went back to her comment about "enema" and asked, "So a doctor will be coming in to administer the...ah...procedure, right?"

Little Jen said, "Procedure? You mean the enema? Nope. Just me! Carrie here will, like, assist me if needed."

"You...ah ...are both going to do this? Um..."

"Yep, we do this all the time! You'll be finey fine!" she said, like we were going to drink a vanilla Coke together. "Just turn on your side—yep, right on your left there—and we'll get started." Carrie immediately left the room, which was smart.

I was taken off guard. Jen wasn't at all the person I had expected to be executing the procedure, or...to be frank...poking around in my ass. I looked at Jackie and Zachera with the expression of: One: OMG, this girl is probably in middle school!! Two: This isn't really happening. Three: If it is happening, you both better wait outside because all hell's going to break loose shortly!

We had waited long enough and the emergency room thing was thankfully behind us, so there wasn't any backing out now. It was just that I had pictured some old, 270-pound, garrulous guy with a beard walking in carrying a bucket, not Jen, the winner of the Illinois Miss Young Teen pageant, and her assistant Barbie. These two teenagers were going to take care of this? Maybe it was just me, but Jen was chewing gum and popping it, if that gives you a clearer picture of the situation and who I was dealing with.

We're not totally sure if what happened made an indelible mark on Jen and her assistant's psyche or not. Maybe they both did an about face regarding their career choice afterward and went into accounting. On the other hand, maybe they never blinked, were totally unaffected, and were secretly thinking about sexy forays with their boyfriends when my personal Hoover Dam exploded. As I said, we're not sure, we don't know, and I'm not calling or Googling them to find out.

I told Jen my stomach hurt, I didn't feel good, and my head was pounding. When it looked like liftoff or detonation time, Jackie and Zachera slipped out the door, saying, "We'll be right outside." Jackie had a twinkle in her eye, looking at me as she went out the door. It seemed to me like my wife and daughter were giggling because they knew what was going to happen and had seen who was going to do it. They wouldn't have giggled, but...still.

I wasn't laughing. This was going to be crazy and wasn't as pictured in my head. Jen—Miss Teen—brought a portable toilet around to the other side of the bed. It was a tiny toilet seat on a plastic tiny frame with a huge garbage bag hanging below it. It looked like it was made for a kindergartner, sort of like a toy, like something you train on.

After Jen set the plastic toilet down off to the side of the table I was sitting on, I surveyed the situation. This was messed up. I'm thinking *Holy Shit !!* I'm sorry, but I couldn't help it. I looked at her incredulously, "Um...Let me get this. You—not a doctor or nurse—are going to do this?!"

"It's all good, don't worry a bit. Let me read the rest of the instructions on this sheet to you."

"Read the rest of the instructions on this sheet'? You're doing this from an instruction sheet? Have you ever done this before?!"

"Oh, like tons of times! No prob!" Jen said, beaming.

For the record, if for any reason you think this wasn't all that embarrassing, remember, I have nothing on. Nothing as in no clothes, no underwear, no gown, just me and my plain bare ass. Parts flopped all everywhere and I was spread out like a frog in a biology class experiment.

At that juncture, I was facing away from Jen, and, at least for the moment, she couldn't see my...ah...um...all my...um...expressions. Jen started right in without hesitation, "Alrighty, you need to curl your legs up so you're in a fun little ball. Kind of like a chipmunk, ok. Right when you curl up—I'll warn you when—we'll try to insert this enema up your anal canal as far as we can."

"You're going to try?! What happens if it doesn't go in?" I exclaimed.

"It always goes in; don't be silly!" Jen giggled.

The last thing in the world I was being was silly.

Jen continued, "Ok, so this solution will do its job if you really hold it and hold it. Squeezy, squeezy! Then, when you can't hold it any longer and feel like you might burst, I want you to quickly jump off the table, get to our cute portable toilet over there and let it all go."

I couldn't believe she said, "squeezy, squeezy." I countered with, "Sorry, but I can't jump off of anything at this point."

"I know, I'll help you. We'll make it to the toilet before everything lets loose…if you can hold it."

"If I can hold it? What if I can't hold it? Or, what if nothing happens?"

"Oh, it will happen. It's just a matter of when. Hopefully we'll make it to the toilet!"

"Hopefully?"

Jen didn't respond and started reading her instructions again out loud. In her fun cheery way, she said, "Ok!! Let's do this! Let's put this puppy where it needs to go! Scooch up more, ok. Remember! Hold it tight as long as you can, at least ten seconds! We'll count together, ok? You have to make it to ten!"

I couldn't believe this was about to take place or what was going to happen at the point of attack. Judging from how many days I had been holding everything back, we're talkin' major tsunami. What if it blew her back against the wall? What if it blew me off the table? What if nothing happened? What if the toilet bag hanging there in that feeble plastic stand wasn't big enough? OMG…this could be a colossal mess!

Cinderella continued, "Now curl your legs up tighter. Tighty tight!! Now, stick your bum out towards me." There, I was sticking my bum out. "The longer you hold it, the better it will work and we won't have to do another one."

"Another one!!"

"Yeah, well, your chart says you reallyyyy need this enema, Mr. Emmet. So, if this doesn't work, we'll just keep trying."

I started to say, "What if..." but before I could go on, I felt this tube entering my ass. It started getting deeper and deeper and Jen yelled, "Fire in the hole !!" and she shot some vile concoction up through the tube!

It hit me like a Ghost Pepper! "Holy crap! Holy shit!" It was like instant! "What the hellll!!"

Jen yelled, "Hold it! Hold it!" and started counting! Ten—nine—Arrrrrhh!!—eight—seven—It was like a wet paper towel trying to hold back Niagara Falls! Six—five—OMG!—four.

"Aaaahhrrrr!! I'm not going to make it!! OMGGGG!!" I screamed.

Jen kept yelling, "Hold it, hold it!!!...three...!!"

I bellowed, "I...can'tttt hold!" @#$!"

Jen shouted, "Holdddd it!!"

That was it!! I couldn't stand it any longer. It was the next reckoning. Off the table and heading for the tiny portable toilet, I was a Boeing 747 airliner trying to land on a helicopter pad. "AAAARRRHHHH!!! I'm not going to make it!!"

Jen yelled, "I've got you! I've got you!!" and somehow guided me to the portable toilet. I was "coming in hot!" with no seconds left.

What happened next I won't go into, but it was a damn good thing they used stretchy garbage bags! It went on and on. Luckily, Jen had conveniently made like Elvis and left the room, leaving me to—privately—take part in the longest orchestral movement in the history of symphonic music.

After the War of the Worlds ended, I tried to get up and get my underwear on, caught my foot in one of the holes and slammed into a blood pressure stand. Quickly putting my hand against the wall, I saved the damn thing, but immediately got caught up in its tubes and cuffs. Finally, after getting untangled, I sat down, tried to catch my breath, and got the rest of my clothes on.

Meanwhile, back at the ranch, Jen had evidently called Carrie back for reinforcements. Carrie bopped in to help with a lollipop in her mouth and said, "How'd it go?"

I'm not kidding. They had been instructed to transport said toilet bag out of the room to God knows where. They each grabbed a handle, pulled up, grunted, looked at each other quizzically, and set it back down. It was too heavy! Thankfully, they tried a second time and somehow got it sliding towards the door. I didn't know it, but they passed right by Jackie and Zachera sitting on the out-side bench. Zachera told me later that two girls went by, kind of duck-walking and trying to drag a sagging garbage bag down the hall. She said both were looking as far off to the side as they could.

Evidently, after the armada went by, Jackie said Zachera turned to her and said, "Mom, was thatttt from Dad?" They walked quizzi-cally back into my room in amazement. I looked up and sheepishly said, "I feel better."

21

Recovery Revisited

Em slept in today. He got up at ten in the morning, which he never does. He's got a lot of water around his ankles and lower legs. A couple of weeks ago while he was being tested, they gave him a drug called Furosemide, a.k.a. Lasik. They think it will keep the water in his legs down. I hope. When I see him like that, it scares me. I don't want him to start having heart problems, too. He said he had headaches all night. He ate half a bagel with cream cheese, awful coffee, couple spoons of Activia yogurt, and a bit of banana. He doesn't eat much. I went for a walk by myself and wondered when we would ever get back home. Texted my friends and ate lunch in our room. Took vitals, did blue/green breathing exercises. Guy nurse came to do what Em calls "the Egg Thing" because the steam that comes out of the machine smells like rotten eggs. Really hates that stinky one! Tried to walk, move, shuffle to the bathroom by himself. Took a long time, but he made it. Did all his breathing tools throughout the day. He felt like trying to attempt the arm exercises they gave him. Tried to stand up and balance on one foot, but it was hard. He lifted his knees up some and then attempted to squat but that was a no-go, to say the least! But as he said, "At least it's something!" He's being so positive, and he's smiling like the Em we know! – Jac

Recovery is a substantial concept. Thoughts heading into my transplant seemed simple. *Get a transplant—live or die. If it's live—work to recover.* Straightforward, not complicated. Bam! 'Tis what you do.

Sort of...Not so fast, pilgrim.

The best way to explain what happened during my recovery period is a "Hints and Tips" sort of section. Taking you through each and every tedious day might cause you to immediately drop off this book at the Salvation Army. Hence, here are some important, handy dandy tips to help. I've culled out the exceedingly boring ones for your reading pleasure. Whether you are recovering from a serious health issue, going to the local casino, or betting on the Kentucky Derby, the following tips will help. Trust me. There's something to be learned with every step we take in life.

During my recovery phase, please remember the transplant team's extremely honest and signature adage: "You are trading your lung problems for different problems." Of course, it would be wonderful to go back to the health you had when you were twenty-five, just like it would be great to get back the $100 bill you placed on Buttocks the Wonder Horse at the derby. But, as things go, you can't. Life changes, and if you received a transplant, you have new, miraculous lungs, or a new heart, or a couple of kidneys, or any of the other organs transplanted today.

William Shakespeare's character Friar Lawrence offers a life view to Juliet when she's despondent. He offers her some good, positive thoughts and then adds, "there art thou happy." It's the same today as it was over four hundred years ago. You have reasons to be positive. You are living, you're with people you love, so "there art thou happy." Go with it! You are living with problems you can deal with. If it was 1950, the doctors would be talking to your next of kin and calling a priest. Want to go back to a time when you couldn't breathe, or are you ok with taking a million pills a day? "I'll take the pill door for $200, Bill." It's all perspective. We choose our perspective, and that perspective is totally up to you, and you only.

Want to relive having an oxygen tube stuck up your nose and the stress of knowing you're reaching the last level? Or, are you ok with mild incontinence and loads of pills? If you've chosen to live, repeat the bottom line: "Living is better than dying." It's not always true, but it is most of the time. This platitude kept me going through tough times, believe me. Is it harsh?—yes. Is it the truth?—yes.

Someone reading this may say, "Yeah, but Sam will have Gretchen and the rest of the family to help." This sounds like a grand plan at first, but at some point, these people need their own lives. At some point you will have to start doing things on your own.

At first, yes, you need help, lots of it. It's pretty obvious when you can't do a damn thing. When Gretchen hands you a glass of water and you pour it in your ear, it's help time. But, at some point during your recovery, you need to take the reins. You need to perform these necessary duties by yourself. Remember, eventually you will be able to; the time will come. I remember the day I said to Jackie, "I'll take care of my meds from now on." She gave me a surprised look. I said, "I mean it. You've been ordering all these drugs, setting them up for me, making sure I take the right ones at the proper time of day. I need to do that now. I'll order them, set them up, and take responsibility for them." Jackie helped me with so many things, I knew she really appreciated me taking on my daily task.

Sirloin Tips

What would comments about lung transplants, other transplants, or life be if they didn't offer tips? I mean, we read cookbooks with all sorts of tips for grilling or getting lumps out of gravy. Our cellphones advertise recipes for everything under the sun. Keep in mind, these tips aren't just for someone engaged in a lung transplant or severe surgery of some kind. These tips work for everyone because life is just f—— crazy and you never know what's coming next. Tips help with kite flying, ice fishing, bocce ball, directions to the museum, and mosh pit etiquette. Never ignore tips. We all need tips. So, where to start?

Let's begin with pills, and then move on. I know, I know, you're thinking "I don't need to read about pills," but you do. Why? Because pills are going to happen and you're going to be up close and personal with them at some point. Fine, if you live in Peru, never took a pill in your life, and are 115 years old, this section might not apply. But, if you're like everyone else, you might need a pill here and there. If so, here're some tips. What if, for example, you miscount, get the wrong day or month, take someone else's pills, or, my favorite, mistakenly spill your pills all over the floor with your dog gobbling them up, making his ears grow five times their size. I'm just sayin'.

Pills

No matter what operation or wild thing the doctors did, inevitably you will be involved in all sorts of pills. Whether you have gangrene or a strange looking case of jock itch poking out your underwear, pills are the thing. Pills will not be a choice. Look in the mirror. You want to look better than that.

Mr. General Public says all the time, "It's terrible how many pills/medications people take these days!" To which I offer, "Yep, we ought to go back to the good ol' days when they gave you a swig of whiskey, strapped you to a blood-stained oak table, and started cuttin'." This is not heading into a debate on the use/possible misuse of pharmaceuticals. Yes, it's an important issue and bad things have happened by overmedicating, it's just that—for medical use only—the saying "better life with drugs" works. If it weren't for miracle drugs, well...you get the picture.

One day whilst laying on a small bed in my favorite hospital, I came up with an idea. It had nothing to do with pulling something out of my throat or messing with a tube, but it did have to do with the friggin' 3,457 pills I had to take per day. Alright, a bit less, but my thought was, *what if I can talk my doctors into less pills? There's no way I need thatttt many per day!* I casually suggested to my lung team, you know, off the cuff, "Hey, ah...I was thinking, nice day, eh? Yep and...ah...so I'm thinkin'...how about we just drop these three big pills here? You know, these bright green ones the size of a cucumber? Like, not take them?"

A futile attempt. My lung team gave me this blank look and said, "You mean those big, bright green ones that are...keeping...you...

alive?" It was like the gangster movies, "Forgetttt about itttt! Ain't happenin', pal!!"

Trying to get confidential with the nurse who handled my pill orders, I said, "Mary, can I talk to you about my pills, you know, just you and me? No one else, you know, cause I have been skipping those heart pills that make my joints hurt. I skip one or two a week. Not all the time, so no biggie, right?!"

Mary said, "Do you do this with any other medications you're supposed to take?"

I thought, *Ok, at least she's talking to me about the idea.* I answered, "Well…ah nope…just those pain-in-the-ass achy ones."

Mary moved on with other questions, like how I was doing overall and if I was eating healthily. Then she left saying, "See you next time!" all happy and cheery. I thought, *I'm in the clear on this one. Score one for Mr. Patient!*

It wasn't more than a minute before Kristen opened up the door without even knocking. "Robert, Mary tells me you've been skipping your heart medication pills?!"

Jeeeessszzzz O'Mally Pete's!! You can't get past these people! They are so on it, so don't even think about it! For the record: I'll admit they're on it so you stay alive. Besides, that's just the nurses and PTs. If your doctors found out, they'd yell, "Take the pills and shut up!" (Of course, they don't yell and would never say that, but you know damn well they want to.)

When Kristen, my nurse for life, uses my first name before she says something, as in, "Robert! Listen to me," I'm usually breaking a rule and there's no use in even debating. It's a done deal. Case closed. She's really serious. She doesn't do the mess-around.

Kristen really is my nurse for life. The hospital told me that. I was like, "For life?" and they said yes. Which was pretty cool, I'll have to admit. But then I thought, *What if she quits and becomes a dancer on a cruise ship or something?* Kristen said that wouldn't happen, so I stopped worrying about it.

So, ok, there're going to be pills. They started me off with about forty pills per day. Yes, that was a cupful—literally. But, after you start to get better physically and put some time between you and your surgery, many of the pills may not be needed. Your pill numbers diminish. One day, someone like Kristen will walk in on your appointment and say, "Em, we're going to stop taking the round red squiggly pill from now on."

"Oh really, why?"

"Well, because it was a pill that kept your gallbladder from instantly deflating like a pricked balloon and shooting all around inside you. But now that your gallbladder is fine, there's no need to worry about that happening."

"Oh...ok," I said, thinking there was something slightly off about the balloon image. It was best not to ask. Probably, in truth, the real answer was so complicated they chose to make something up like the balloon/bladder story, which they probably created over morning coffee. As in:

Nurse 1: "We've got to get Patient Q to understand the importance of the pills he's taking."

Nurse 2: "Let's tell him there was a guy who skipped his pills and his penis started shrinking."

You're expecting me to say, "Ok, they'd never do that," but I'm not going to. These nurses are tough, salt of the earth, down and dirty, nasty in a good way, seen everything there is to see, touched things that would make your skin crawl, out-on-the-streets indestructible. Do you think for a minute they wouldn't talk like that over coffee?

I'm almost three years out since my transplant; I'm down to about eighteen pills per day. In all seriousness, it all comes down to the statement they keep repeating, "Having a lung transplant is exchanging one health issue for another. It's just that with the latter, you live." Like I said, they don't do the mess-around.

There's no sense in the staff telling you everything is going to be rosy, because that's not reality. Considering what surgeons have to do to transplant someone else's lungs into your body, it's a modern wonder you're not in some Plexiglas Smithsonian exhibit. To expect you will be back bowling next week with your team The Bowling Stones is a bit, shall we say, dubious.

Whilst depositing my meds in their plastic daily cubicles one morning at our breakfast table, an older family member stopped by to say hello. He came in, I got him a cup of coffee, and we chatted about the day's events. While watching me slowly drop my pills into their proper plastic holders for a minute or five, he said, "You know, Bob…taking that many pills isn't good for you."

I raised my eyebrow and laughed, "Well, if I don't take them…I'll die."

He quickly moved on to a different subject. "How 'bout those Detroit Tigers!?"

All in all, taking pills every day hasn't bothered me. In the scope of things, it pales compared to other more difficult procedures, of which I will not go into. It also doubly pales compared to trying to breathe when you can't. Another "case closed."

As I mentioned earlier, the Shakespeare/Friar Lawrence deal, "There art thou happy." It's the same "Romeo is alive. There art thou happy! U2 is coming to Chicago. There art thou happy!"

You are living, you are around people you love, you can order pizza, drink beer (later on), grill stuff (without getting in the smoke), try on clothes at Sidewalk Sale Days (with latex gloves), or have your grandchild go on a walk with you. It's a process you can live with—pun intended. So what if your grandchild asks why you're wearing a mask over your mouth? Tell her you're getting ready for Halloween. She'll believe you, and it beats the alternative…every time.

Your life comes down to things like this: would you rather try to feebly shuffle slowly into a restaurant pulling an oxygen tank, or endure mild incontinence in the restaurant restroom? Would you rather have a breathing tube up your nose 24/7, knowing at some point it won't be enough oxygen, or take lots of pills each morning and night? I took the latter in each case, and I'm sitting here looking out my den window at a beautiful fall day. Your viewpoint changes; that's all I'm sayin'. You have to be happy because taking pills is, for the most part, pretty easy comparatively. More importantly, you have to be happy because you're attending your daughter's wedding.

Tip—your pills are mega important. First, it will take your doctors a while to figure out the exact dosage for each med: med = pill... as in, "Did you take your meds?" At first, they will monitor you like an astronaut, checking oxygen levels, blood draws, skin tone, urine samples, and your bank account. It's all good—go with it.

Learn the names, shapes, and colors of all your meds. This is difficult because, to start with, they give two different names to the same damn pill—generic and some Latin deal (see upcoming rant). They do the same thing with outdoor plants, which tells you where you stand in the hierarchy of things.

This is how I got to know my pills. Tevia, in *Fiddler on the Roof*, says in his deep growly voice, "Sounds crazy, noooo?" Unless you have a photographic memory, start by learning the size, shape, and color of each pill before trying to memorize their inane names. You think a pill's name is pretty easy to remember and elementary, but remember, you're starting all this whilst high on major narcotics. When a seven-foot pink bunny hands you your pill box some morning, you'll understand.

Each pill's exact name will kick in once you see them over and over. Early on, your mind is going to be zooey, as I said, so just be The Dude and say, "Far out, man!" to everything and do what people say. Keeping pills in one particular order and taking them the same way each day really helps, too. Trust me, the weekly plastic trays, cubicles, square-holder thingies keep you sane. You'll ask, "What day is it, honey?" You laugh now, but it gets like that.

Soon, the blurriness gets better. Life will stop looking like a fogged-up mirror. The zany narcos will fade into the sunset and you'll start saying things like, "Hey, I know you! You're my brother!" But, after taking meds morning and night, day after day, monotony sets in. You'll begin thinking, "Did I take my meds?" You won't tell anybody because you sound like *One Flew Over the Cuckoo's Nest* and you don't want to end up like the giant Indian guy. You'll get so familiar with the process it will become second nature. You won't focus on it; you'll take your pills robotically, which causes the problem. You're saying, "Aw, that won't happen to me," but it will. It happens to everyone. Therefore, here's a plan to fight it.

Set alarms on your cellphone—two alarms in the morning and two in the evening (depending on when you take your pills, etc.). Set each morning alarm fifteen minutes apart, so if you miss the first one, you'll be reminded again. The same with the evening. If you have trouble programing your cell, ask your daughter or son to show you—different generation. If you're vain and insist on doing things on your own, get over that shit in one big hurry!

Get a plastic, seven-day pill separator. Fill each day with the correct meds. You can fill each day with the incorrect meds if you want, but you'll be asking why you look similar to the Wicked Witch of the West. I fill my pill holders on Sunday mornings. For some of us, it's a lifelong crucial chore whether we like it or not. Subsequently, you need an orderly system.

Get a quality water bottle with at least a one-inch nozzle and a pop-open spout that works well. You're going to partake in this maneuver, hopefully, a million times (think about it, eh?). Struggling day and night with a hard-to-open top makes no sense. BTW—clean all water bottles frequently, like once a week. It's not hard: put them in the kitchen sink with warm, soapy water, slosh them around, and rinse with hot water. Two minutes, tops. If you don't clean them, they get full of whatever and you don't want to intake "whatever."

Get to know your pills. When you go back to the doctors, your nurse will immediately ask you what pills you're taking. It's embarrassing to say, "You know, I flat out have no idea." Start with size and shape. "The pale-yellow football one is Mackeraltummysodastream—'take once in the morning, once in the evening.'" As I said, forget the name at first. Specific pill names will come to you later when the walls aren't talking to you.

Here's a good way to take pills. I won't go into bad ways, but the guy in the bed next to me tried throwing them up in the air and catching them with his mouth—pills all over floor, nurse not happy. He was on the narcos I mentioned, so…Become an artist at swallowing your pills. Hopefully, that's the only place they need to go!

Always handle pills in the same order; it quells confusion. Follow the damn directions. If you mess up on the time thing, it's ok (in most cases) as long as you take them within a reasonable period. I asked one nurse, "What if I forget taking my pills by a few hours?"

The nurse answered, "Hour, two ain't gonna kill ya." Nurses get right to the point. Bam! Got thangs to do!!

Here's how to take pills. I'm not you, I know, it's just that I've been invited to the National Pill Taking Championships in Hoboken, New Jersey, twice. We're all different, but try my New Pillow (just kidding). If you think you're flawless at taking pills, skip this little ditty. If you hate taking pills, gag, spill pills all over, or the whole damn thing is just a pain in the ass, try this method:

You might be saying, "OMG…I can't believe he's actually telling me how to take friggin' pills! Anyone can do that!!" Fine. Do you know how many patients say taking their pills is their number-one problem? You don't, so just read this. Besides, I made this exceedingly short just for you:

One: Pills and water bottle in ready position on stable table. You don't do wobbly. Swig of water to wet your mouth so pills don't stick like peanut butter.

Two: Put number of pills you're comfortable taking at one time in hand. With mouth open (kind of a must) in one motion, toss pills to the back of your mouth like you would a handful of peanuts. Towards the back part only. Don't go goofy and throw them in haphazardly. They stick.

Three: Immediately tilt head back, take robust pull of water from water bottle nozzle, swallow firmly, sending pills and water down your throat. No wimpy swallows! Those who hesitate are lost. Whoosh! Right down! If you're timid, things get screwed up—get yourself set and go for it!

Voila! Pills go right to your stomach, all safe and sound. Drink more water to complete task because water is good for you. These steps take practice—especially for those who can't even handle peas—but you'll become a pro in no time. BTW—your hands might shake from meds like Prednisone, etc., so take your time and focus. As Arnold says, "Uuuu con doo eeeetttt!"

The above are suggestions. If they don't work, at least I tried.

Regarding your mental state/life/pills, I had mentioned a rant about pharmaceutical companies and their stupid names:

Rant

This is written in rant format…every word is being yelled and may contain expletives. Needs to be read that way. Out loud is even better:

Pill companies make shit up! They confuse the fuck out of everyone on purpose—even the Russians—with their dumbass names!! Pronounce and listen to these ridiculous names slowly—names like Alwaysventammusilate, Extrafistofmarmalade, Yomommasittightacuss, Zeg, Germomomoland2, and Fixaflat. Don't bother Googling these. If companies don't screw you up with their stupid-ass names, they make some up with no vowels at all—like TRXZICXZT . "Yes, miss, I'm next in line and need a refill of TRXZICXZT."

"Excuseeee meeee, sir, what did you just call me?!!"

"No, no! It's just this stupid…never mind!"

How about naming something "XZXZXZCCVVCCVVV." How's that for no vowels? It's a pill for greedy executives and can only be taken on their yacht.

Andddd…while I'm at it, what's with the list of side effects?! "Gerballygobzone may cause warts and loss of fingertips." WTF?!! I'm sitting watching the evening news—which evidently only people over sixty years old watch anymore—and ads try to convince me I have diarrhea and constipation (at the same time), a limp dick, and mush for brains.

Another insane ad starts by listing side effects first—brilliant decision by some dumbass ad agent: "If you take cherry tasting Blopperzippyrzol, you may experience vomiting, death (my favorite), your right foot falling off, and the famous black slippery discharge."

What the hell!! Yep, tomorrow I'm running out and buying some of that shit!

Black slippery discharge?! Where does this discharge come from? The local sewer outlet? There are a number of orifices on my body that can discharge. My skin discharges sweat, so does that mean black ooze will come out of my arm?! That'd be great at the beach. "Hey, honey, pass the white hotel towel, I've got some black slippery discharge coming out of my arm. Oh, and I'll have another tuna sandwich." Is discharge a fun word (?), and what the hell does "slippery" have to do with anything?! Does that mean if the discharge gets on the floor, someone may slip on it like a banana peel? Is that why you're warning me? Cause it's slippery? Maybe I could mix it with my BBQ beans recipe? "Man, Bill, that's some good tasting, slippery beans ya got there!"

WHO IN THE ____ MAKES SHIT LIKE THAT UP?!!

Do ad executives sit around at goddamn lunch saying, "Phil, listen, let's add black slippery discharge to the list of symptoms we're inventing. It'll liven it up."

Phil, "Do those pills really do that?"

Stanley, with his Chucky-looking face, says, "No, asshole, but they'll never know!"

Maybe they could legalize a product that will give you all of those side effects at once! You know, get it over with! Why don't they print on the label, "When taking this product, you'll experience euphoria, orgasmic pleasure, joy, love, a drunken mind state, and incredible bliss!" Bliss would ——ing sell better, wouldn't it?

Rant over.

To be fair, even though there're some bizarre things about pills, you need them. Until the medical field comes up with magic fairy dust or "Beam me up, Scotty" tubes, you'll be taking pills the rest of your life. Along the way, you will get foggy/forgetful regarding whether you took your pills or not. You're saying, "Rightttt, that would never happen!" but it will. Remember what I said above:

Cue the pink bunny. You were on a lot of narcotics, experienced excruciating pain, or lost some memory due to being under during surgery for a week or something. So, it's kind of like your cellphone going on the fritz—you might recover some of your info, but you're not getting all of it back! Getting older doesn't help the situation any either.

Even if you're boppin' around eating Hostess pies and checkin' out your hot yoga instructor, it's human nature to forget your routine when things get routine. You'll think, *Did I take my morning pills?* You'll get so familiar with your pill process—day after day—it will become second nature. You'll start to take them robotically and then start missing your meds here and there. Then the mind games: *Ok. I took my morning pills. I know I did. Yes, I did. Maybe I didn't. Wait. I'm not sure. Did I?* (checking pill bag). *Yep, I did… But was that yesterday's set of pills?"*

My daughter put med alarm times on my cellphone. (I didn't know my phone could do that.) And, while we're on the subject of conspiracy theories, why is it that every garden-watering wand dribbles? We can go to the moon, but we can't make those wands stop leaking like something else I know and am up close and personal with!

Side bar: *Lasagna Tips*

This sounds ridiculous, but it's important. If you know you're having surgery ahead of time, make up the following signs or have your support group make them. There's a good chance you won't be able to talk right after surgery, or the hospital drugs make your sentences sound like heavy metal music played at a slow speed. Trust me—make these signs:

I'm hot = I'm way damn hot! Perspiration's dripping down my face from the ten heated blankets piled on top of me!

I am cold = Ditto, in reverse.

I have to go to the bathroom = Ol' Johnson down there is temporarily out of order and acting strange, so you may get wet. Ever changed a male baby's diaper? Cold air = Niagara Falls. It might be worse for females, I don't know. Does it all go in the same direction as ours??

Ice chips, please. = Nurses give you all sorts of reasons why you can't have water. But…wait for it…you can ask for more ice chips! Not sure what the damn difference is between ice chips and water, but keep asking for more and they keep giving them to ya!

There's a bedpan under my ass = (Alternative sign?). The hospital staff tries to communicate, keep notes, do things in order, but let me tell you, nobody is perfect. Occasionally, especially after procedures, the staff goes on break, changes shifts, or moves to Canada. Whatever. Unfortunately, the bedpan they stuck under your ass… is like…still there. You can't remove it because it contains a massive tsunami that came out your ass. They left it there and you fell asleep. Shift change, no one knows, and your ass, and said bedpan, have now become one solid item. A cable and winch are now needed for removal.

I love you = Please make this sign. You'll want to say this to the ones you love. It's a bit different "I love you" than when you both go off to work. It will be wayyyy more important than that. Again, trust me, make the sign.

Making six simple signs isn't difficult, and calligraphy's not necessary. It's a small, yet quite vital task.

Then, there's the shower. You can try to rough it and not take one, but pretty soon people won't be able to stand near you…or your sheets.

Interesting staff trick #23:

Nobody wants to move any body part/thing/whatever after surgery. Nope. Nohow. No way. Therefore, getting you to take a shower is used as motivation to get you out of bed, moving, and eventually walking.

I know, you're saying "What about a sponge bath?" Ain't the same thing—gets pretty intimate, things happen, all the rubbing, etc. I passed on the sponge bath. Declined. Therefore, due to my reluctance, I now had one choice: taking a real shower. A real shower comes in two packages. One: A nurse, not necessarily the same gender, will take a shower with you because you'll need help and probably can't stand up worth shit. When my nurse/PT told me she would get in the shower with me, I was shocked and thought, "Yikes!" because, as I've already mentioned earlier, doing so could create one elongated problem. Speaking for my gender only—male—when you get turned on for any reason, shape, or thought, it shows. Prominently, right there kind of thing. Knee jerk reaction without the knee. I'm just sayin'. Girls think guys have total control of this situation. They're all, "Well, you don't haveeee to let that happen, you know!" Like many things in life, that's is a myth. "It" has its own mind.

If you're a guy, you remember being in seventh grade. Of course, this would neverrrr happen…when your nurse, who's in your shower, washes between your legs with warm water!? Drugs or no drugs, listless or full of energy, I'm telling you, it's a problem. Then, when the nurse tells you she's done this "hundreds of times," wild mental images show up like Stanley Kubrick's *A Clockwork Orange*. But, in reality—come on!—they've seen humans before, no big deal.

After all that, at some juncture, you'll get the green light to shower by yourself. That's when you'll say goodbye to your shower-nurse friend and figure out how to move your body from bed to shower. First, don't pop up in the morning all bright and cheery, ready to make pancakes. This is progression. Progression should never be taken for granted. Start slowly and tell your left leg to move slightly to the left…explain to your right leg there's no arguing…left shoulder moves on an angle…right leg slides toward other leg…right arm tries to push against propped-up pillow, which doesn't work…pillow falls off bed, spilling cup of water with special bent straw…water on floor is slippage problem…bit by bit, try to sit up…breathe for a while…think happy thoughts…when no happy thoughts show up…think about giving it a go tomorrow…or continue arm pushing to no avail…swivel legs further to the left…stop…swear…think about hitting the call button…suck it up, don't hit call button…get feet on floor…wait thirty minutes.

Your journey across to the bathroom gets even better and will take far longer. Step by step ("slowly he turned") you get there, you put your hand on the bathroom door molding…and wait another thirty minutes.

Getting close to or in the bathroom with buckets, tubes, and your rolling stand has been thought-provoking in more than one way. Now, try to get through the bathroom door. Not as easy as you thought, but you get in with your whole entourage of equipment clanging and dangling. Do the shuffle maneuver to get in position near front of shower. Problem/roadblock: how to take off dumb blue gown with ties in the back…hmmm? Hold on to handy-dandy chrome handle on wall. Pulling gown over head is out. Showering with gown on could work, but it will eventually become a clingy lifejacket. Reach behind nightgown and find wet, totally knotted strings. Semi-forcefully rip strings completely off gown. With gown loose, wiggle until gown slides off shoulders and pools around ankles. This may or may not work, depending on body shape or how wet you got it from the shower or incontinence.

I really disliked calling my hospital apparel a "gown." It's a strange word. It's like "from." If you say "gown" or "from" by themselves, they sound goofy. Try it. When you're in the hospital, a gown is necessary—I see their point. But they're demoralizing because your butt is hanging out for all to see, and wearing a nightshirt to bed is just weird because I never use one. My dad did. The one with the gray and white stripes, like the scrawny old guy moving down the spooky castle hallway with a lit candle.

Anyway…taking a post-surgery shower by yourself is risky, at best. Here's why.

One: Until you're really ready and your partner/nurse gives you the "A-Ok," do not attempt taking a shower alone!! If help is around—family, nurse, someone down the hall, or an available physical therapist—maybe give it a go.

Two: Only attempt a shower if your balance is good. It won't be. If you can't get to or into the shower by yourself, there's a pretty good chance showering alone could be a disaster.

Three: Don't spray the shower stream directly on stitches. Force of habit will cause you to forget and screw this up. Use your Frankenstein voice, "Spraying hot water on stitches—noooo gooooouuud!"

Four: Know where the shower handles are and make sure you can reach them—even with soap in your eyes. This is a must! Imagine: No one around, you fall down in a heap on the tub floor, and can't reach the handles. A beached whale comes to mind. If this happens, there're a lot of colloquial words or phrases to shout, or just use the old standby that rhymes with "mitt."

Five: Move—under control. No fast moves. A shower is not a timed event, unless you're using coin slots. Make sure someone is within earshot.

Six: Feelin' woozy? Grab shower handle and wait thirty seconds. If it doesn't get better, call for help and stop taking a shot of whiskey before your shower.

Seven: If a shower just ain't happenin', don't worry. Your nurse's arsenal contains sponges, mops, towels, hoses, squeegees, siphons, etc. Besides, your wounds are covered and clean, so the rest of you can smell to high heaven. Let them deal with it—you're dealing with enough. Let yourself go!

Important item: In-shower chair. You laugh, but they work. Watch it though, they're tricky. You might not be able to stand up very long, if at all, so a shower chair is a must. Don't just grab any chair; it won't work. First, make damn sure you know how to work your water temperature valve. Sometimes an errant plumber reverses the cold-water/hot-water line by mistake. Find out BEFORE you step in and jump a foot high because the water's one degree from ice. Jumping is bad. Don't jump for anything. Do not jump. No jumping. You have tubes coming out of everywhere, IVs in your upper arm, bandages in certain areas, a catheter you know where, goofy narcotic vision, cotton up your nose for some reason, a slippery chair seat, and whatever can tangle or twist the wrong way will. This all adds up to entertainment.

Case in point: Attempting to take shower seated on your handy-dandy shower chair with soap on ledge—you try to scooch chair to reach the damn soap, which takes muscles that used to be attached to something—"shit"—rubber knobs on the bottom of the overly safe shower chair won't scooch—again—"shit"—on your way to being a prune, you reach for the soap a littleeee bit harder, causing your left stomach-tube to pull out—don't try to stick it back in!—a third "shit!!"—while catching the flailing stomach-tube hose spewing whatever, soap gets in your eyes and you now can't see—you mistakenly step out of the shower, slipping awkwardly on the wet tile floor. Read my lips: This can not happen! We're talkin' way bad.

Anddddd...if you're thinking this will never happen, well...okie dokie.

Eventually, you'll figure it all out because you'll take your time and make it work. My first shower took fourteen hours. Alright, maybe not that long, but felt like it. When I finished and somehow wrinkled my way to bed, there was a full lunch tray on one table and a full dinner tray on the desk, if that tells you how long it took!

You are saying, "Yeah, but someone would help." Not always. Your family won't be there 24/7. Uncle Herbert's been drinking your Royal Crown all afternoon, the call button doesn't work, and the hospital hallway is as silent as a circus tent an hour after the show's over. Don't worry, they'll eventually have a grand opening for their newly renovated patient rooms and find you there—fossilized.

Also, once you semi-master showering alone, watch out for hidden problems. Post-surgery, whilst taking a shower, I decided, like always, to shave. I proceeded to cut myself with my completely safe Gillette razor. Normally this was no big deal, but because I was taking major blood thinners, when I looked down, it looked like the shower scene from *Psycho*. Blood everywhere!

I yelled to Jackie, "Houston, we have a problem!" She came running in, threw open the shower curtain, and screamed, just like in the movie!

My chin was fine...after a while. Soooo...take your time with everything, be more careful than you've been in your past life, and follow directions because your nurses really do know what the hell they're talking about!

22

Patient vs. Caregiver

His pain med was lowered. Fewer milligrams. Straining to use the bathroom is causing chest pain, especially around his chest staples. MiraLAX is now his friend. He's really worried about his swollen legs and ankles. He's trying to use Tramadol, which is not as strong as Norco, but I don't want him to suffer like this. I know he's not telling me how bad it is. Two more tries on the blue-and-green breathing machine. Insulin test at twelve midnight. Maybe he'll do better tomorrow. Slept on his side for most of the night. Needed pain meds earlier than scheduled. I think he went through a lot the last two days—more than he's saying. More MiraLAX. Tests all day. Found a new blood clot. Not good because they already found two old clots in his lungs and some in his legs. Took a nap. Long day. – Jac

The lung-team doctors were particularly happy with my progress and continually urged me to exercise and follow instructions, of which there were many. During days of healing and getting stronger, my hospital appointments started to dwindle from two a day, to once, to every two or three days. Then, after good reports, appointments were scheduled once a week. As time passed and I was a year out, as they say, journeys from my hometown, Boyne City, to Chicago took place every one or two months.

When my next clinic or lung transplant team meeting appointment date showed up on my calendar, I would check to see if it coincided with Mr. Paul's lung transplant forum (the Mr. Paul's forum I told you about earlier, which has no relation to Mrs. Paul's Fish Sticks). These forums took place every month on Wednesdays, and patients living somewhat close to Chicago could, luckily, make each one. My trek was farther and involved many of hours of driving, gas money, and sitting, so, unfortunately, some of these fruitful encounters were missed.

One month, after morning appointments at MMHMMM, I finally made one. Mr. Paul's forum didn't have a speaker that day because the doctor scheduled to talk to us about lung transplant longevity had been called into surgery. After introductions and reviewing the rules, as always, Mr. Paul led us into discussion by asking if we could talk about what was on our mind. What questions we had, what thoughts and ideas had been running around in our head since the last forum. It didn't take long for people to jump in with comments, and our hour-and-a-half forum was off and running.

There was a concept/debate/idea discussed that particular day that was important. Important not only to patients and their family/support givers, but as a study in family dynamics and differing viewpoints.

The subject dominating the discussion revolved around "the patient" and "the caregiver"—what worked, what didn't. How things went, how they didn't. There were caregivers in the room sitting next to their patient to help deal with downtown Chicago traffic, parking, or just the logistics of getting through the myriad of elevators, crowded hallways, room numbers, and coffee stands. These caregivers came to listen and learn, as well.

One family sitting together in the circle had come to the forum because their relative was in the midst of all his qualifying tests for a possible lung transplant. They were scared to death about what was happening all around them and very emotional. What they said was extremely interesting because we all knew what a scary situation they were in. We had all been there. They talked about dealing with guilt.

When a patient goes through something as traumatic as a single- or double-lung transplant, or any highly dangerous surgery, their specific viewpoint on life can change. It may not; we're all different, but the overriding commentary from the transplant patients in the room was that after surgery, they looked at life in a completely different way. Things that seemed so very intense and important before were now minor. When you weighed almost dying against a petty argument with a neighbor or an errant bill mistake, suddenly, said arguments paled. Family differences that had always escalated now seemed small and inconsequential.

Because of this viewpoint adjustment, many patients said, "You know, all I want is for my family to be happy. I don't want them to fuss over me, to worry, to have to do things for me, to have to come see me or get me something."

One recurring patient comment surfaced: "I don't want to be a burden to my family." Being a burden was the last thing patients wanted. Many didn't want visitors because they knew how difficult it was for family to take work days off, to travel to the hospital, to park downtown, to have to spend money. They wanted their loved ones to be happy and to continue with their lives, not disrupt them.

I, personally, asked for no visitors other than Jackie, Zachera, and Ryan. Someone in the group asked me why. My answer was, "Well, alright...first of all, I'm going to look like shit with tubes coming out of me from my nose to my ass. It's not that I'm vain, it's just that I'm going to be a hot mess. Second, if I request no visitors, visitors won't have to disrupt their lives to come see me. If I make that request, it takes the onus off them. It'll make it easier for them, which is what I want. Why in the world would I want people to fuss over me, take work off, buy stale chocolate candies, and find some kind of parking blocks and blocks from the hospital, just to sit in a germy, stuffy hospital room and watch pieces of pepperoni pizza flow through my feeding tube? I wouldn't. I'd be happier if they called me or sent funny GIFs. No in-person viewing of my procedures, no watching me get shots, no wondering why I was breathing into weird vials, or having to ask, 'What was your transplant like? Did you ask the doctors if you could look at your old lungs and stuff?' Also, what if I was in the bathroom with the door open and visitors walked in with my stupid blue gown open all the way to China? Hmmm? Nothing like tubes, mile-long scars, and purple skin to brighten up the mood, eh? What about the monitor going 'blip...blip...blip' with my heart rate? I could secretly slide my hand down the side of my hospital bed and unplug it. It would stop and they'd all jump up like 'OMG'!! Then, I'd plug it back in to resume the 'blip...blip...blip' and say, 'Hey! Just foolin'. Don't be so jumpy!' and they'd all be pissed off but laugh—uncomfortably."

Ok, I'd never pull the heart monitor plug out like that. Funny idea, though, but not cool. It's just that I didn't want people to fuss.

If you think about it, this viewpoint makes perfect sense. I mean, here is this patient lying on a bed who's just been through the ringer, gauntlet, and lawnmower at the same time. A patient who's mustered up all the strength he or she had deep inside to physically and mentally get through such traumatic surgery. Here is a person who has clearly looked death in the face with only a fifty-fifty chance of surviving such a massive surgery as they entered the operating room's swinging doors. The last thing this patient wants—after all that—is to worry about burdening others. To be honest, they just want to be calm, lie there, and get better. They want to be as still as they can. Just lie there. In short, not deal with anything else. I mean it. In many cases, that's it. They've been through so much, by all means throw in some family arguments, a brooding teenager with green hair and a quarter growing in her earlobe, or grandpa exhorting how much good the NRA does for our country. It's like Greta Garbo, "they vont to be aloneee."

By design, this thought process, this patient viewpoint, worked and made sense. But...nobody bought it.

It was like everyone had to act like they always do in the movies. Someone's sick in the hospital, so we have to go visit, sit around, talk to them when they're barely awake, and watch the nurses do stuff. Is that helping or making someone feel better? Wouldn't it be better to leave them alone with just their closest people? Couldn't you just call them and let whomever is helping screen the calls? How about sending something you know the patient likes with your name on it? That works. They'd know you were thinking of them, which is all you can really do. You're not going to visit and fix someone's bandages or wrap them a new cast, so just chill. If a patient really, truly wants company, so be it. But, more often than not, at that point, they don't. It's like having a baby; every single relative from here to Alaska has to come see the baby an hour after you just had her. What's with that!? A close friend put out a one-week moratorium on the "coming to see the baby" thing. They decided they wanted the first week their child was on this earth all to themselves. One relative said, all huffy, "Can you imagine not letting us come see the baby, for goodness sakes!" Please, some-one take her out in the back forty. The relative, not the baby.

In our lung forum that day, "feeling guilty" became an intriguing and worthwhile topic. Many of the caregivers and support friends who were there spoke up and said, "But, I want to help in any way I can. I have been married to my husband for forty-three years. I want to get him whatever he needs, do what he needs, be there for him. I have a family to care for, but he comes first."

Another caregiver said, "It's not a burden to help or be here. I would feel terrible if I couldn't." One of this person's family spoke up about guilt, "I haven't been able to help all these years because I don't live here. I live across the United States. I wanted to help, but I couldn't leave my job, my family. Since I couldn't be here for her, I've felt terribly guilty. I wasn't here for her; I should have been."

What became clear was there were two viewpoints from opposite sides of the spectrum about the same subject. The patient and caregiver both wanted to help the other, to love the other. Patients expressed the need to not burden their family, to not have them fuss—because they loved them. The caregiver/family/support people wanted to be there, to ease the patient's pain, difficulty, and angst—because they loved them.

With all of this, what was the true problem? The pervading issue turned out to be: what both sides wanted for the other was exactly the opposite of what was actually needed. Here's the conundrum in its simplest form: Patient—"I don't want to be a burden, "vs. family—"I want to help." It was the Red Sox vs. Yankees because of their deep love for each other.

You might think this conundrum sounds crazy. Or, you might say, "Yeah, but...does this really happen?" Well, ok, it does happen. Many of the patients in our forum talked about it at length. It happened to them. It happened to me. There are so many instances in life where this happens: Do we make people happy, or do we unknowingly make things worse?

The last thing I wanted was to have my daughter lying awake at night wondering if I was still breathing. Her viewpoint turned into angst. Angst all over the place. My viewpoint: I'm so lucky to be alive, I'm busting with happiness! We loved each other and I wanted her and everyone around me to be happy...because I made it through, I'm living.

We are all here, alive. It's a brand-new day! Be happy! Be worried about me? Hell, it looked like I was going to be dead six months before, and now I'm living, breathing, talking, riding my bike down a beautiful northern Michigan forest path with Jackie. Think about it. Why in the world would I want someone to fuss over me now? There was no need. I made it! I'm wearing the Life is Good t-shirt! I'm on the NFL big screen yelling "Hi, Mom, send money!" I am the No Worries, Life is Grand guy; I'm the Beach Boys' Kokomo melody, "Palm trees in the sand"; I'm sayin', "Everythin' Irie, mon'"; the Miller High Life ad: "Living each day to the fullest; the full Monty big time! Why? Because I made it back!

As it turned out, my daughter was at the other end of the field, the other end zone, the exact opposite. Zachera loves me, didn't want to lose me, and was scared. She had come so close to losing me she now felt the slightest problem that showed up would send me back to the operating room or do terrible harm. I don't blame her. The whole shootin' match was dangerous, tenuous, and life threatening—a lot to take in when you're twenty-five and an only child.

Zachera woke up every morning with the reality that I could die any second. Her fears were legitimate; she had listened to what the doctors said during recovery. She knew the percentages, statistics, graphs. She knew there were issues lurking in every corner and, knowing me, I probably wouldn't pay attention to many of them like I should. She was haunted by the feeling she wasn't doing enough to help me; there had to be more she could do.

Later on, after talking to her at length about her feelings during that period of time, Zachera said, "All I could think about was, *I need to be at the hospital.* I thought, *To hell with my job, I need to be helping my dad.*" She added, "I felt I was the only one who could make you do all the right things health wise—eat right, avoid dangerous foods with mold like blue cheese or mushrooms, lose weight, exercise more, wear a mask. I knew Mom was helping, but wanted to do more, to buy you books on how to survive in your condition, get you to use hand sanitizer every five minutes, climb more stairs, wear your mask in the shower, wear your mask every-where." She felt she was the only one who could get me to do my breathing procedures correctly and became obsessed with why I wouldn't try harder after being given donor lungs, a new life. Why wouldn't I follow my health rules more closely, go to the other side of the street if people were smoking? She wanted me to live so badly it hurt.

Moral of the story: Understanding what's best in certain situations is a tough road, but the key is, everyone walks down it differently. In retrospect, like all things in life—it's a compromise. As each patient told their story, the forum group came to the conclusion that loving each other was the most important thing of all. Just loving some-one superseded all else. That maybe the best thing to do was walk next to them, not in front of them.

Maybe asking a patient what they need is more important than telling them what they need. Realize, even if it is against all your instincts, you don't have to be out in front paving the way. Let the patient pave their own way—with your support—with you by their side.

Letting a family member fuss some might be ok, too. Maybe they need to fuss, to do their part, because it's the only way they can show their love. A family member might want to feel that at least they did something for you after they left your hospital room. It's not easy feeling helpless when the person you love is lying there.

Tricky turns.

Life can get complicated. We can't make everyone happy all the time, but maybe we can make someone happy some of the time. What's the rule for family relationships, caregivers, support friends? Are there any? Maybe it's no rules—just love as much as you can.

23

Ethics, Judgment, Dying

Walked from the hospital to a restaurant called Yolk, a good breakfast place close by. Slow going. We stopped along the way two or three times for Bob to rest. Sat on a granite wall and talked until he felt ready to go further. It was a nice morning and being in downtown Chicago is so interesting—a far cry from our little town. Afterwards, he couldn't stop talking about how good his breakfast was. Finally, I said, 'Alright already with the breakfast!!' We laughed. Daylight Savings Time, EST vs. CST, is messing us up regarding Em's pills. Mike says to stay with one time regarding pills. Consistency is important, but one hour isn't a problem unless it's before a blood draw. I try to keep notes. It's all complicated and stuff. He drank Kionex…sp? 120 mL to lower potassium level. Thursdays he takes extra Vitamin D and calcium. Wonder why only Thursdays? – Jac

This turned out to be a tough chapter to write. Difficult because it deals with dying, judgment, ethics, and mysteries of life—just a few light issues. Getting close to death elicits images of dark-cloaked beings, floating tombstones, sickles—does death always hang out on a wheat field?—and going across rivers, for some reason.

One specific river was named Styx. In Greek mythology Styx is a deity and a river (at the same time?) forming a boundary between

Earth and the Underworld, a domain ruled by Hades. A rock group picked up on this whole death and dark deal and named themselves Styx. In the days of heavy metal with high pitched guitar shrieks and lots and lots of screaming, Styx had album covers featuring stylized death symbols and paraphernalia. Seems appropriate, I guess. Or not. Also seems like all the written words, pictures, and speeches ever conjured up by people somewhere in time about death all melted into the same bizarre metaphor.

Myths/metaphors like these help some people. I don't know. People like stories that make them feel good or restored about death, that put life in a birthday box. Kind of like a good mom or dad trying to make their daughter or son feel better by buying them ice cream after something bad happened.

Little boy says, "Goin' on that roller coaster isn't going to be good, Dad, I'm scared."

Dad replies, "Don't worry, son, your mom will take care of your underwear when you get off that Rip Your Ass Off ride. It's like Moses climbing Mt. Sinai—uphill, lots of gravel, sandal slippage, no water, but…everything will be fine." So, on it goes.

When people are confronted with death, it makes them nervous and jittery. It's a finality we've all tried to get straight in our minds one way or another but never can. Death makes people stop their lives for a minute and reflect. It's pretty difficult to avoid and such reflection can be confusing, very confusing. So, it's just rough at every turn, which is why so many people, groups, churches, and organizations toil at dealing with it so diligently.

I'm not sure why everyone avoids looking at the full cycle of life. It's part of us. *The Lion King* musical has a song which explains this circle and makes you feel better, until you leave the theatre. You could listen to it on the radio, but it wouldn't have the same impact. No matter what you sing or say, people still sort of make like it will never happen to them. People watch news reports about hurricanes where trees have flattened homes. The news reporter standing in the rain says, "And three died in the home behind me. Back to you, Dave." Then, people get up and grab another Bud

Light from the fridge and check Sunday's football scores. They're not going to think about it. Who wants to do that?

Three months or so before my lung transplant, MMHMMM's team told me I had around nine or ten months left to live. It was a shock, but the strange thing was, I wasn't afraid of dying. I really wasn't. This was mentioned earlier, but it would be good if you knew how that strong belief held up through everything. It did hold up, and helped me continually as I tried to survive. But later, looking at the same thought after I made it back out through those infamous surgery doors, my view of dying took on a different slant.

When it became clear my lungs were failing and things were going downhill quickly, I was backed into a corner. There was no way out. It was dying in nine months or having a mammoth lung transplant where the odds of survival weren't the best. The thing was, though, it really wasn't an option. What kind of option or warranty ends right after you make it? Like soon. Dying in nine months was no option. This may sound crazy, but it was easy to come up with "Ok, no option, so I'm goin' all in." I mean, what else was there to do? In my mind there wasn't any other way to think about it: Do I have the transplant surgery they're talking about, or die soon? I remember thinking, if door number one—transplant surgery— there had to be 100 percent commitment. One hundred percent. It felt like, *Really? Does picking 65 percent make any sense?* For me, it was "you're in or you're out." There was no in-between. I went all in, my doctors and family went all in, and I now live each day as a magnificent gift.

After coming through my transplant so well, my viewpoint on death changed slightly. Not much, but enough to mention. My new slant on this fathomless subject of death is, I'm living and want to keep living. I'm still not afraid to die and still feel at peace with my life—a life that's been lived fully. It's just that now there's this sly side bar: All these wonderful people worked so incredibly hard to keep me alive, so many supported me and gave me the undeterred love I needed—I don't want to die soon and disappoint them.

Jeeezzzz, life always throws a curveball when you don't expect it!

Alright, not one person who went through being part of it all would be disappointed. They would never feel that way. They would learn from my situation and keep getting better and better at saving people's lives in the future; my support family would have an even deeper understanding of what love really is. It's just that now I feel like I owe everyone so very, very much. I don't want to let them down. When my back was to the wall, I was like, "Let's do this!" To be perfectly honest and cut to the chase, now that I'm back, I don't want to leave.

Having these feelings might seem completely ridiculous, but life is so powerful the thought of letting down the people who gave my life back enters strongly into the equation. The whole thing was so large it can never, ever be, "Oh, well." My being here has become its own entity. I was ready to let go, to die, because there was no other path. I actually thought I was being brave, but looking back on it, is being backed into a corner bravery, or simply baseline survival? Now that I no longer have IPF in my body, now that I'm strong, I have a choice, a choice that's very important to me. The doctors worked so hard and diligently to save me and then I die a few years later? I don't want that to happen. My family went through tough, tough times because of me and then I'm not around anymore? Somehow, I feel like if I don't keep living, I'll be a Christmas present no one wanted—a nice thought, nice try, but taken back to the store. I mean it. Now I have to live to make all the angst and toil worth it.

View of dying—no change. Wanting to make everyone's work worthwhile—big change. Of course, then there's a new problem: What if I don't live for a long time? What if I'm doing great and some stupid ass runs me over while looking at their cellphone? It's like, well, that was a waste of time and energy. Having that happen would keep me from keepin' on keepin' on, and there are special patients out there who own serious stock in that saying to let it fritter away in the wind. It's a phrase that keeps people strong; it must not be taken lightly.

Maybe I'm perseverating on the ill wind Mark Twain famously

talked about, "[that]...will find you when you least expect it and aren't looking." I knock on wood a lot. It's my duty to keep on living. Of course, we want to keep going; we all do, but it's more than that. Now, because everyone saved me, it's imperative to make it in the record books as the longest living lung transplant patient ever. For me, yes. For my family and my doctors—far more so.

This is as honest as I can possibly be. I met one of the longest living lung transplant survivors in the United States recently. She's lived twenty-two years since her transplant in 1996. She was one of the first ever. I gave her the biggest and most deep-felt hug because I was so proud of her and knew what it took. The same thing needs to happen to everyone who helped me.

So, my view now has an aside to my 100 percent deep belief in not being afraid to die. Now I'm 90 percent not afraid, and 10 percent kind of owing in arrears. Sounds a lot like my home mortgage in reverse.

Wrestling with life and death, making sense of it all, is age old. Having been there, been close, should help in obtaining a sense of it all. But only a little. I haven't been able to comprehend having transplanted lungs, let alone death. Maybe things will sink in and I'll have a sounder view. I don't know.

Death is touchy. First of all, it's almost incomprehensible when you're just out walking your dog or eating a baloney sandwich. Look at how people act at funerals, for instance. Everyone gets all weird and spooky. For one thing, there's a casket in the room with a real body in it. That's a bit different than shopping at the farmer's market or going to a Halloween parade. There are these oversized, wild bouquets; a strange man whom nobody really knows standing at the entrance greeting people with a pursed smile; a book to sign for some reason; the church lady making things tidy by dusting—which goes right along with the dust to dust metaphor; and mints. Always mints.

All my life, I've hated going to funerals. Not because someone died, but because of the way people act while at the "showing." OMG, they actually call it that! Now there's a term that elicits negative thoughts before the funeral even starts to rev up. And thennnn, they have a "wake." Really? "A wake," "alive,"—"Hi there!?" Interesting, and just plain-ass weird.

Perhaps you've noticed funerals have mood changes. First everyone is quiet and somber, walking around, not looking anyone directly in the eye. Then the service starts and if someone makes a slight sound in their pew, everyone turns and gives them the eye.

As for the word "pew," Jake says, "What's that thar new wooden bench ya made there, Willy?"

Willy ponders, "Don't know. Guess I'll call it a pew."

Jake exclaims, "Hey! I've got one: 'He who farts in church...'"

Willy frowns, "I know, I know. Already thoughta that one."

Who made up the word "pew"? And, who specifically assigned it to churches?

Finally, after the service ends, here comes the mood change. The serious person you met at the door now has a big smile on his face and directs you to a party. Maybe "wake" means "Let's get chipper." People wake up. Everyone is laughing, telling jokes, and talking about the deal they got on their new car. It happens every time and seems so fake. Like, we went through the motions, so let's shelve the death idea and start networking.

How weird is it? People standing by a box with a dead body in it saying, "He looks so good." Would you really say that to someone who just lost a loved one? That he looks far better dead than he ever did mowing his lawn? Also, please do me a favor and never, ever ask someone, "How are you holding up?" This was voted number one in *Fun & Travel Magazine* for the stupidest question asked at funerals. "Ah, there's a handrail, so I'm holding up, not down." Dumbass question.

Alright, that was harsh, but we need to get better at this funeral thing. At least show up and try to help, which is the important thing. But don't say dumb stuff.

It's just that sorrow is singular. There is no right way to handle having someone you love die. Don't ever let someone tell you how you should feel or act when it comes to sorrow. People who use the "should" word are invariably judgmental, terrible human beings. This also goes for what you believe. Some people in this world truly think it's their lot in life to get people to believe what they believe. I think it makes them feel safer. Believe me, their way of thinking isn't the only circus in town and there's a giant difference between sharing beliefs vs. telling someone what they should believe. Some are actually brainwashed into thinking they got the golden ticket and you didn't. Don't even get me goin'.

Sorrow is also solitary. How people deal with their personal sorrow is as private as it gets. Yeah, let ol' Uncle Dooser tell you how to feel (major sarcasm).

The reason not being judgmental is so important to me—and to this book—is because dealing with another person's lungs in your body, or any type of transplant, can bring about judgmental opinions even when it's no one else's business. Up pops another adage: "Opinions are like assholes—everyone's got one." Did you ever wonder why these adages have stuck around so long?

After undergoing a double-lung transplant, I am living. I have lived going on three years—quality years, precious years. Could anyone even think for a fucking second I shouldn't have taken part in a transplant? That the donor didn't want the one they loved to live on in a metaphysical way? Could someone actually believe the religious idea that their god, living in some mythical cloud, told them a transplant was a sin against nature? I'm not going to say another word about people like that. They don't deserve words.

Saving someone's life is such an enormous undertaking to get your head around. I still wrestle with it every single day. How it happens is mind boggling. The fact that someone died, was a donor, and you now have their organ inside you is too big, too difficult, and too much to comprehend. No doubt, issues regarding stem cells, human transplants, and cloning are complicated. People take all sorts of weighted sides—until they need one. Somehow needing a medical marvel to stay alive changes their belief system. Hmmm.

I've asked people with such opinions who they love most in the world. After they think for a minute and tell me, I ask them how they would feel if the only way their loved one could go on living was with a transplant. Would a transplant be ok, then? Or, would they turn it down and let their loved one die because of their supposed beliefs? Tricky turn, those beliefs. A loaded potato.

Since my transplant, different people have actually told me my surgery was very unsettling to them. My initial reaction was, "Excuse me?!" held out for a second or two. But, listening incredulously, they said their god was all-knowing and had his plan. ("His" plan—interesting. Women create life, but god is a "he.") Then, they told me "his plan" doesn't include doctors transplanting human organs to save people. Their god somehow gave surgeons the ability to successfully transplant or do stem cell work to save human lives, but won't allow it. Wow...getting pretty sketchy here. God's doing stuff, but then not doing stuff.

Ahhhh, the plot thickens, though, because their plan can conveniently change when they want it to. When I asked, "What if it was your own daughter?" their eyes shifted, and after stammering, they answered, "Well, my own daughter...ah...well, that's different." You betcha it is.

When this particular incident occurred, I almost asked the pompous hypocrites if it was ok with them if I ate my sandwich. You know, with my miraculous, but blasphemous lungs breathing and all... but...I didn't. Valuable time should be used on helping and loving people, not on shortsighted, judgmental thinking.

My parents taught me at a very young age a person's beliefs are their own, and, other than crimes that hurt other human beings, I should never judge. "What a person believes is their business, not yours," I can hear my mother saying. I probably could tell you where my mother was standing in our house and what she was cooking at the time. It was at an age where figuring it all out was important, you know, when you thought you could. I asked her a theoretical question, "But, Mom, what if people are wrong?"

"Well then, misterrrr (doing her impression of John Wayne), who are you to decide whether someone is wrong or not?" I enjoyed having these conversations with my mother. She was smart.

I came back with, "What if someone hurts someone or kills someone. Don't we judge them?"

My mother replied, "Good question—complicated, but good. Take too long to answer before dinner. Wash your hands and go get your father in the garage."

She wanted to tell me her thoughts, but I was two years old and holding a teddy bear (kidding). Ok, twelve, and maybe the subject could wait.

I waited. My mother never passed up a chance to make a point, though—she was Irish. After a pause and a stir of a pan, she said, "Look, I'll just say this. Some things in our world are inherently wrong: From the beginning of time people had sense enough to know murder, lying, cheating, or hurting someone was wrong. We all know certain things in the world we can't allow. Do people who do these things always get caught? No. But, we as a society must honor basic principles of right and wrong. Go get your father." At least she didn't say, "Ask your father." My mother was good like that.

"But what if someone believes what they're doing is right, when it's really wrong?"

"Listen! Last words! Dinner is going to burn." And with an exasperated look, she said, "When you get older, people in your life who aren't smart will tell you what's right and wrong, but they don't know any more than the lamppost down the street. They are people who believe in myths, not truth."

Dinner was good.

24

Visiting the Children's Hospital

Pretty good morning. He's sleeping longer, much more than ear-
lier days. He did stairs today. He was so proud of making it up one
flight! He said, 'I went all the way up and back down! Ok, it took me
fifteen minutes, but I did it!' He laughed. 'National speed record!
I'll have to call The Chicago Tribune...ha!' I love hearing him laugh.
Met with Dr. Aisner, who deals with infectious diseases. I didn't want
to sit in his waiting room one minute longer. Infectious diseases—
ick. Bob says Dr. Aisner is an interesting guy and they talked about
top restaurants in Chicago. This morning he walked more stair steps
than last time. He's so proud of that. So am I. – Jac

Children's hospitals and my double-lung transplant? Because
after you know what it's like, the whole hospital/death/health/heal-
ing process takes on a much different hue.

I met wonderful, needy, and beautiful children at MMHMMM. My
transplant recovery took time before, between and after. Because
MMHMMM is huge, has about one thousand wings, harbors
unusual looking departments, and spreads out over half of downtown Chicago, I went for walks within the complex.

The area where Paul held his lung transplant forums became
familiar and was right next to MMHMMM's Children's Center. I had
visited a children's hospital in Grand Rapids, Michigan, when my

daughter, who was thirteen, had a life-threatening accident and was saved by—once again—incredible doctors. While there, there was time to walk around and, if lucky, meet wonderful, cheery children. Cheery despite their difficult situation. It had been incredibly sad and uplifting at the same time.

Now, here was another children's hospital with young people in the same boat. With all my idle time, maybe I could stop by and talk to a few of them, maybe help brighten up their day. Paul from our lung forum hooked me up with some close friends working in the children's hospital wing and I was given the chance to meet some of the children whose health was being ravaged by cancer or other maladies, as long as it was safe in my condition and safe for them. While there, all I could think was, *they are so innocent.* Incredibly innocent. Life was throwing them an awful curve, an awful blow. Making it through a double-lung transplant needed strength and I had to put powerful resolve in my head. These children had only been on this earth a short while. How could they have possibly gained the life tools it would take to survive their ordeal, to endure?

One child had been in the hospital for over a year. She was eight years old with bright blue eyes and beautiful long light-blond hair with one partial side shaven. A younger boy stood next to her, holding her hand. He was small, maybe four years old. The young girl said, "I'm Arielle." She knew what to say and seemed like she had met other people this same way. Arielle dropped Jimmy's hand, turned, and said, "I'm ten, and he's Jimmy. He just got here. His parents said he has what I have, so I take him around when I go for a walk. I show him stuff." Jimmy nodded, but didn't say anything, just looked up.

Arielle—of course, it would be. Fantasy probably helped. She said, "Come on, let me show you. I know this floor pretty good 'cause they won't let me on the elevator to go to other floors without my mom or a nurse. There's lots of cool places here, though!" Cool places...in a hospital. She took my hand, pulled Jimmy by the wrist, and off we went exploring.

I could tell you about our whole trip around the fifth floor, the nurses Arielle introduced me to, Marty, who took care of the monitors in her room, the exercise equipment she made me try—she liked the bicycle with moving handle bars the best. She knew what door led to staff supplies, but made me promise not to tell.

After looking around, we dropped off Jimmy at the nurses' station, where his nurse was waiting quietly to take him for his procedure. We waved goodbye and headed down to Arielle's room—room 507—accompanied by Sara, her nurse. Arielle had decorated drawings taped all over her walls, and a giant box of Crayola Crayons. Her art included a turkey she colored last Thanksgiving, Mickey and Minnie Mouse bright and smiling, and a big farmhouse. She had pictures of young guys in rock bands taped all over. One was autographed, and I asked if she had met them. She said, "Na, my dad got it for me. They're cool!" There was also a picture of her mom and dad on a stand next to her hospital bed. "I can make this bed tilt and go up and down. It's like a Disney ride I can ride on over and over—but don't tell the nurses!"

After talking to Arielle for a while and finding out her favorite music, TV shows, and movies, I said, "I've got to get going, but it would be nice to visit you again if you would like." Arielle looked up at me and said, "My mom and my doctor think I'll get better." I paused, thinking hard about what she had just said and holding back my emotions. Reaching under my jacket lying on a chair next to her bed, I pulled out a plastic bag (so much for wrapping). It was a gift I'd bought for her at the hospital's gift shop on the main floor. She pulled it out, saw it was a teddy bear, and yelled "Yea!!" She jumped off her bed, gave me a big thank-you hug, and said, "Wanna see something neat!?"

"Yes!!" I said, feeling the magnitude of what her parents and doctor had told me.

Arielle went over to a dresser where she kept all her clothes and pulled on the big, bottom drawer. It stuck some, but when she got it all the way open, sitting there were six of the same teddy bears! I said, "Oh, gee. I should have gotten you something different."

Arielle immediately said, "I'll name him Robert. That's your name, so it will be his. They all have names and I get them out every night so they can play on my bed. We have great parties!"

We all need teddy bears, just in different ways.

Introducing you to Arielle and Jimmy is significant because they are all the children in all the hospitals in the world. All of them. If you've never walked through the corridors of a children's hospital cancer ward, or any ward, it's special—and not the special you might be thinking. If you visit one, you'll be very, very surprised. You will be next to the strongest sense of hope you will ever experience.

You will be taken back, amazed. Their moments are not sad. They are made up of what will happen next, in the future. They know not of sadness; they haven't been on Earth long enough. They are tomorrow, not yesterday.

I'd like to ask you to do something for me. Take one day out of your life and visit a children's ward. I'd dare you, but we don't know each other that well. Most people don't take time out of their lives to visit any hospital, let alone one like Arielle's. I mean, why would you do something like that on any given day? But, think about it. How many hours/days have you spent sitting on a couch watching some other human being play sports? How many hundreds of minutes have you spent reading cellphone news about gloom and doom, or wandered aimlessly around a mall? What if just for one day, one hour, you did something unusual, different. You certainly don't have to, but—at least one time—one single day—what if you visited a children's hospital and bought a child a bear? Maybe only once, but it would be something you actually did one day.

The children are there.

You don't have to know someone in particular. Google the nearest children's hospital and ask how you could visit a child and give them a small gift. The hospital would love to set it up and will understand what to do. It's far easier than you'd think. If you know a doctor, they can set you up as well. Believe me, they have connections. The hospital will know what child could really use a lift, something fun in their life, even if it's just for a short while. Even if it's their sixth teddy bear. It will change your perspective on things, I guarantee. Maybe you're thinking, "I could take one morning out of my life to do that." Or...?

Our culture relishes its stars, its famous people. That's fine and all; we know their names really, really well—but we don't know the names of the little boys or girls who are fighting to stay alive in that hospital you drive by every day on your way to work. We don't know the names of extraordinary doctors and staff who live near you or me, who never get noticed, never get media attention. The nurse who helps Arielle every day; the teacher who helps a student grappling with his parent's divorce; the policewoman who puts her life on the line to save someone in a burning car. We don't know who they are. Their names. Did the media post their pictures? Probably not, but we need to.

A few years ago, there was a fairly obscure article in the *Detroit Free Press* about a young doctor working with a top cancer team at Wayne State University in Detroit, Michigan. He was thirty-six years old and in the news because he was robbed going to his car one evening and shot dead. This doctor was considered one of the leading researchers on cancer breakthroughs. The article said, amongst other things, his yearly salary was $80,000, which caught my eye. We pay stars millions and millions per year. This year, one baseball pitcher in the National League was paid $203,000 per game, which totaled $9 million for the season. The cancer specialist, whose cure might have saved millions, got $80,000 per year? Are we crazy? Will people look at us in future history books like complete idiots? Will they say, "Whattttt were they thinking?!" Why would you pay someone a million dollars just to cure cancer?

I'm afraid this section may sound preachy. I didn't want it to be. I just wanted to suggest buying a child a teddy bear and handing it to them in person. After having your life saved by extraordinary people, you gain a new perspective regarding who's a superstar and who isn't. It shouldn't take a life-ending illness to realize the superstar isn't the running back on Sunday TV.

So, this is sort of a take it or leave it proposition. I probably won't be inundated with emails saying, "OMG, I took your advice and visited…"I understand if you don't want to visit a children's hospital; there are many semi-legitimate reasons not to. Maybe in years ahead you might. You can seriously think about visiting someone, or forget the idea and go get a pack of cigarettes. Just please know you can make a huge smile appear on the face of a child who is walking around a lonely hospital ward. A smile for someone who truly needs it—if you want to. A perspective change can sometimes change your perspective. Your values, priorities, and viewpoints will change. There will be reset—it will be good—and then you'll walk back out of the hospital doors into the sunshine.

But what usually happens, from what I've observed over sixty-eight years, is people move along in their lives doing normal things. Normal days go by. We never think about getting really sick or dying. We go our way with a built-up, false sense of security. I did. We don't go there—we don't want to go there. We don't think about it because we're doing fine and we believe life will stay fine. Life is for the living. But sometimes people have their normal lives interrupted. A list isn't necessary here—too many to count. Health issues arise. Maybe small issues attended to at home—a cut requiring a bandaid, a bruise, or a bad cold. Maybe bigger problems crop up and you see your local doctor. Then, your doctor might send you to the hospital for the day or you even have to stay overnight, checking things out. We know things happen, but ignoring is easier than confronting. Sometimes people get really sick and die. All of a sudden, we become distinctly aware, go to the funeral, pay our respects. After a few days, we go back to not thinking about it. Maybe it takes a while. Maybe not.

Given all the above, why would I ask you to take a visit to a children's hospital? It's not episode six of some Netflix series. It's real, though, and we can't ignore what's going on around us all the time.

This is not a plea to fix all the problems of the world. It's just good to have some cognizance of what's happening in that building you drove by yesterday. Why do people who volunteer say how much they enjoy it and how good they feel afterwards? Interestingly, one university study found people who volunteer live longer. Another said people who volunteer continually say they're happier than they were before they started volunteering. Am I making this up? No. Ask someone you know who volunteers at your local food bank; homes for battered women; organizations that help people, like the Lions or Rotary; or the uncountable people who help their neighbor down the block. As I said, the children are there, and they're probably not going home soon.

25

Famous Children's Book:
Everyone Does What??

Made it through the night with just Tylenol. Very, very big deal. Had a great morning. Bought the sunhat they said he'd need because of his low immune system and strong sun rays. His voice has been weak. He's concerned that his voice cuts out. Wonder why it does that?...He's smiling because it's Happy St. Patrick's Day! He wants to try to walk all the way down to the Chicago River because the city of Chicago turns the Chicago River green! It's environmentally safe because they're treating it for algae, and since their process happens to turn the river a vivid green, why not do it on Paddy's Day! I don't know if Bob can walk that far, though. There're an awful lot of people out and walking around, too, so I worry about him catching something. He has a lung bronchoscopy at 4:45 p.m. Hope it goes well, fingers crossed. He hates bronks because he feels awful for days afterward. – Jac

All sorts of weird things are going to happen to your body once you've had one of the myriads of procedures they've come up with to make your problem better. It's kind of like your car. If your car slid off the shoulder of the road, hit a tree, and you were able to somehow get back on the road and drive away, a funny noise or some kind of clunk might show up as you drive along. It's the same with human beings. When we metaphorically hit a tree health wise, weird things happen—your ears droop, your belly button pops out, you grow a sixth toe.

Lots of funny noises have been coming out of me since my transplant, let me tell you. Jackie says they're not new and happen every time I eat chili, but I know these babies are different. You can tell. I bent over to tie my shoe the other day and something went "brrrannnng pinnggg" and it didn't come out of the usual orifice. At this point in my recovery, if this sound wasn't followed by me passing out, drooling, or being sent to the ER, I was like, "All good. Whatever."

You are going to hear the phrase "a new normal" a lot. Well, I'd love to tell you it doesn't exist, but—alas—it does. You can't expect all the king's men and all the king's women to put you back together again perfectly. Therefore—and you knew this was coming—you have to take extra care of your body now, even if you didn't your whole damn life. Now, every time I think about slipping up regarding the right thing to do for my body, two things immediately pop into my head. One: my donor family, and, two: how hard my surgeons/doctors/staff worked. This cures me right away. Well, most of the time.

A close patient friend recently called me for moral support. Some patients do this; it's obvious why. She's been going through extremely difficult health issues, some of which are leading to new and dangerous surgery. I told her to call me whenever she wanted, but especially if she got really down. After we talked for a while, I told her I did this private, quiet "just today" thing for myself whenever whatever got extremely tough.

She asked me, "What do you mean you did a 'just today' thing?"

I answered, "You know, during really difficult days, my mind would wander to the what ifs. What if I get an infection? What if I get pneumonia? What if something else shows up in my body needing more surgery? What if I have a heart attack? How am I going to cope or get up the stairs? What if I die? How is my family going to handle all this? And on and on."

She said, "That's what's happening to me. That's why I called you. I'm getting so depressed. Those same thoughts roll over and over in my head. I can't stop them."

I explained to her, "Constant worry was taking its toll on me and I had to stop it. I couldn't keep letting it happen. It was literally killing me. So, I came up with a phrase that would signal my brain to knock it off, shut it down completely."

"What do you mean?"

"Well, the words 'just today' came to me. Every time negative thoughts showed up, I would ask myself, 'Is this something for tomorrow or the future?' If the answer was 'yes,' then I'd say—actually, and, importantly, out loud—'just today.' Nurses would say, 'excuse me?' and I'd say, 'Oh nothing, I'm just talkin' to myself.' But I really did say those words. My life had to be 'just today,' absolutely today, not tomorrow, not next week, not in the future. 'Just today'. It was my way of dealing with all the indecision, wondering, and worry."

"I think I need something like that," she said softly. There was a long pause. "I've got to stop thinking about all the negatives. Rob, I start to think about (I could hear her starting to cry)...I don't know...dying, ya know. I start thinking about all the things that will happen. My family...and..."

I said, "Being in our type of situation brings us much closer to all those realities—realities you've been able to easily keep in the back of your mind, keep at arm's length. They all come flowing to the front. Sometimes in waves." I offered, "For me, saying 'just today' brought me back to now. I had to have it. Sometimes I'd say it three or four times to make my brain focus because it's not easy. It brought me back to the hour I was in, the minute I was in, where I was right then and there. It stopped the tomorrows. We all have to think about the future at some point; it's just that it was so detrimental. I couldn't keep doing it."

She said, "I can't either."

"It sounds strange, but it's kind of like a mantra—like in yoga or meditation. Saying 'just today' makes me track the idea of right now, this second, not where the unknown future lurks. The unknown gets its share of play so I try really, really hard to make today the thing."

We talked about meditation sites online and how they might help. Then we ended and she thanked me. There wasn't anything to thank me for; it was what every person should do when another human being needs help. Talk it out. Help. If you're someone out there who doesn't believe that, well, wait until you get seriously sick.

Hopefully, if you start down the surgery path, there will be time to strengthen your body as much as you can. You are entering one of the biggest battles—if not the biggest battle—you and your body have ever faced. To be completely honest, your surgery is going to take a lot out of you, much more than you think. You want to be as fit as possible going in so your body can take it.

One gentleman I spoke to about his upcoming lung transplant asked me to tell him—truthfully, with no icing on the cake—what things happened to me and what things were different now than before surgery. I felt compelled to tell him and be honest. I said, "Well, I could go on all day, but I want to preface this with 'I made it through ok, so you can too.' The main stuff? The days after surgery were really hard and massively uncomfortable. The drugs helped, but I somehow knew how bad off I was. I couldn't lie down because everything was all about my chest, so I had to sleep sitting up in a chair. That drove me nuts. I woke up often during the night, checking the clock and hoping so hard it was morning. This would happen about every hour or so. Incontinence wasn't fun, either. I had to stand or sit at the toilet and wait and wait to stop going, dribbling, whatever you want to call it. Taking a shower wasn't happening for a number of reasons, but one day my beautiful physical-therapy nurse, who was about five feet one, had long dark hair, said, 'I can help you take a shower.'

I looked at her, surprised, and said, 'Ah, what?...Ah, how would that work?'

'I'll get in the shower with you and help keep you steady and stuff.'

'And...stuff?' All sorts of images flashed in my head, believe me. I said, 'You mean with nothing on?'

She came right back with, 'No, silly, with a bathing suit. I do it all the time in my PT work.'

My reaction was, 'Bathing suit or not, I'm not sure I could handle that! I mean, not handle...I mean...I'd react...hard to explain...ah, not hard...I mean...yeah, well.... ' and we both laughed. She was serious, but so was I!! I mean, Jackie was the one who took care of my in-shower maneuvers! I'm diggin' a hole here. I should stop. LOL.

Lots of normal things became "abby-normal." Showers were one of them. Other things showed up during recovery. Sometimes certain pills made me sick. The lung transplant team checked with me and sometimes changed my dosage or completely switched me to a different type of medication. Patients react to meds in different ways, so they monitored responses constantly.

There really wasn't much discomfort with the stitches across my chest. It was fun to show my guy friends my long scar. It was massive and looked weird. I figured my female friends wouldn't exactly appreciate my big, red, cool scars, but one spoke up, 'Hey! Just because I'm female doesn't mean I don't want to see your stitches!' She found them fascinating...who knew.

Things like sitting up were difficult at best. First, I was afraid I'd mess something up. Make the stitches pop or something, which was truly the last thing I wanted! A whole lot was done in there. I mean, the surgeons weren't playing tiddly winks for ten hours doing nothing. I gradually got better at moving slowly to an upright position and started to feel stronger. I learned I wasn't going to break.

After accomplishing sitting up, turning sideways to get out of bed became my next glorious feat. Thatttt took some doing, but they wanted me up and walking, like you've heard about regarding heart surgery and other procedures. On maybe (pain pills) the third day out of surgery, or what I think was the third day (pain pills), a nurse came in and said, 'Ok, time to take a walk.'

Nurses don't mince words. I started to laugh, 'Walk?! I can hardly move my arm!' Laughing was out, though, because it would hurt! Miss Nurse wasn't laughing. She said, 'Ok, come on, scoot over to the side here.' Scoot...that also made me laugh. Yeah, I'll just scoot over to the side and we'll bop on down to the food court for a salami sandwich. I wanted to yell like Tom Hanks, ('There's NO crying in baseball!!') 'There's NO scooting in this room!!' Crying or yelling, it didn't matter, scoot I did. Ok, she helped me. Seemed to take all afternoon, but we scooted and I actually put my feet on the floor for the first time in quite a while.

Going to the bathroom was difficult and frustrating. You had to get there, figure out how to sit down, followed by 'How the hell do I get back up?!' Like the Netflix series *House of Cards,* there were many crazy episodes that could be listed here. But, during each one, I did what all the patients do—try to survive.

One huge suggestion I'd make to anyone heading into surgery—pre—is to get as strong as you possibly can. Your legs are the most important because you won't be able to use your arms at first. It's all legs. The stronger your legs are, the better you will do. I tried to do as many squats as I could before my surgery. I didn't go wild, but I did try to strengthen my legs. Going up steps, doing squats, stretching, leg lifts all helped later on when really needed. When the time came—after my surgery—my legs were just more than weak, wobbly rubber bands, but what would they have been like if I hadn't worked on them? Jell-O? Beef broth?

Try this: Before surgery or whatever you're headed into, attempt getting out of bed and going to the bathroom with no arms or hand support whatsoever. None at all. Nada. You can only use your legs. Try it. Don't slam into the closet on the way and get hurt, but give it a go. It's not easy. Unless you're a gymnast, you'll be unsteady and have a hell of a time landing on a toilet seat that now looks like a prettyyyy small platform. (Point: Going to the bathroom—number one—standing up, with no arms or hands, can be messy and ruin paint. Therefore, sit down. Sitting down with no arms or hands involved is very, very tricky, unless you have strong legs. Please repeat: Unless you have strong legs. (Guys—make damn sure you don't sit down on you-know-what. Bad, way bad. There's a lot dangling there!)

Ok, so after this minor test, admit it, you're probably not an Olympic athlete. And hmmm, it's possible your surgery may completely disable certain muscles, so if you get corresponding muscles really strong, you might have a fighting chance at movements like sitting up in bed, getting up out of a chair, or standing in one place for more than ten seconds. No matter how many Houdini tricks you have conjured up, you're going to have to go to the bathroom. At present, you trot into the bathroom, do your thing, and never think twice about it.

It's like when you're traveling through Michigan and visit Mackinac Island, the buggy driver tells you a bathroom joke:

Buggy driver drives up to Arch Rock and says: 'Here we have the famous International Bathroom.'

You say: 'Why do they call it an International Bathroom?'

Driver: 'Because when you're heading in, you are Russian. When you get in, you're European. And, when you come out, you're Finnish.'

Even though bathroom problems are not a laughing matter, levity can help, especially when you're in a health battle. You're headed into the Dark Side when it comes to surgery: moving your body, pain you expected, pain you didn't expect, big tubes, small tubes, funny looking skin spots, pills, needles, little gowns with slits in the wrong places, somehow showering, and, our favorite, going to the bathroom. It's reality.

Admit it, we all take our everyday movements for granted—until said movements are no longer possible. Ever hurt your thumb and then try to put on socks or tie your shoes? Same deal. Ever hurt your knee and try walking up steps? Getting as many muscles as strong as possible before surgery will pay tenfold.

Another aspect of surgery such as a lung transplant is dealing with being uncomfortable all the time for quite a while. I told myself before surgery, in one of those private moments when I was being completely honest with myself and not glossing over a damn thing, that the whole mess was going to be tough. Real tough. No doubt about it. And, also, there were going to be times when it was going to be way more than tough, maybe more than ever expected. I had to prepare my mind to get through it plain and simple. If there was going to be a transplant, there was no backing up, backing out, no half-ass. I had to get through whatever they threw at me. As I saw it, it was the deal, the contract: You make me live / I'll gut out what you need in return—no matter what it is. Fair and simple.

For obvious reasons, getting my mind straight in terms of tough-ness/reality hit me when things started to get close. It was the strange denial again. My doctors were talking about the possibility of putting me on the national donor list, all my tests were coming out positive, Dr. Anisee was telling me I was ready, they were ready. It was time for me to stop denying what things were going to be like and start to soul search for real.

Everyone around me, my family, my friends, post-transplant patients at Paul's forums, and my incredible doctors were urging me on, being incredibly supportive. I wanted to live. So, it hap-pened one evening looking out my hospital room window on the seventh floor. Chicago's buildings were lit up and blurred car head-lights appeared below as red and green lines. I sat and thought. *No more questions and no more wondering. I'm going to do this and I'm going to do it 100 percent.* To me it was like stepping onto the field for a championship game. This was it. I had to be strong and tough. I had to step in the batter's box. But it wasn't a game. It was ridiculously more than that.

Making a strong resolve was now about everyone backing me. It was about all the work the doctors had done so far, what they were going to do for me. I felt, right then, at that exact moment, that it was so incredibly big I had to go in full throttle. I made the decision.

Now, looking back, I feel I stuck to my personal promise, my resolve. I tried as hard as I could to hang on, to make it through. I know deep inside I never gave up. It was a promise with no other side. It was stepping up, never out. I also knew it was the only way I would live."

Your mind will control everything. It is absolutely essential to get your mind right regarding what you're about to do. I also felt, at the time, it was only fair to be resilient for everyone else involved. Everyone was in on it. How could I ask them to back me, help me, if I wasn't going to show up on my end?

Hopefully, you know what I mean. Trying to always be strong helped me throughout my life. No matter what the challenge, you had to keep your attitude up. If you did, it helped carry you.

A side point that needs to be mentioned about your body is that this new normal affects things in everyday life you never really thought about. I can't tell you what they are specifically because we're all different, but there will be things you used to do that you blatantly have to stop doing.

My dad always taught me to help out when needed. As he put it, "It's what you do." This usually consisted of helping a friend carry a showcase into his new store; moving a railroad tie to another part of the garden; lifting a 400-pound wood stove with three other guys; or a piano. (What's the damn deal with pianos?! For God's sake, they get heavier every time you look at 'em!) You help out, you just jump in. Wellll, you are going to have to change your ways in one big hurry. You won't want to change, you'll want to grab the side of that newly built, two-by-four wall. But you'll really hurt yourself doing things you used to do automatically.

Remember getting up on your roof to fix something? Remember how the ladder tipped, but you didn't fall? How about working past exhaustion because the job had to be finished that day? You can't pull that anymore because your body is now different than it was at twenty-five. The new normal. Chances are, you'll learn this lesson not because you read this warning section or because of your doctor's directions, but because you hurt yourself and had to crawl back to the hospital. When your doctor asks what happened, you'll say, "Ah, yeah…well…I was…er…we were putting this fairly heavy dock in the lake…and…um…when one of the legs snapped, I…"

I could go on and on about this, but you get the picture. Everyone poops. We're human beans.

26

Friends and Family

Bloodwork this morning. Waited to take meds when he got back to our room. Big appointment today with whole lung team. Should be interesting to hear what they have to say. Will we be able to go home? Zachera called to see if we wanted to meet for dinner. We may go to the Side Door, our favorite place because it's only a couple blocks away. If he gets discharged and we get to go home, I'm going to miss seeing Zachera every day. It's been wonderful to be close to her—albeit in a strange, strange way. – Jac

If you're heading into a transplant surgery, or any major surgery, whether you like it or not you're going to have to learn to rely on your family/friends more than you're used to. You are going to need help in a number of ways, shapes, and forms. It's just the way it is. You won't want to bother any of these people—they have their own lives, their own obligations—but, if you have family/friends like mine, they'll want to be bothered no matter when or where.

This is a "tricky turn," as Maude would say in the movie *Harold and Maude*. There's nothing easy about the whole thing. The same comments show up with every "pre" transplant patient I've worked with. "I don't want to be any trouble."; "I don't want people to fuss."; "I'm not used to asking others for help. I'm the one who helps," which is exactly the point. It's like playing tag when you're "it." Your turn to be helped.

MMHMMM or whatever hospital/doctor/team you choose will interview not only you, but also your family/friends as part of a comprehensive study on whether you will be able to get through the whole lung transplant ordeal. It's that big. It's extremely difficult to understand, at that point, how broad the procedure really is and how important they will be. If you're not quite sure how big, ask your lung team if you can see the booklet they have depicting everything from the beginning to recovery. It's important to look.

This is new territory. You can't possibly imagine everything that's going to happen to you, your family, and friends. At some point, whether very soon or months down the road, you will need them. Who's taking your car back to your home now that you are living in or near the hospital? Who's taking care of your dog or cat? Who's going to gather and figure out what clothes you'll need? Is your house being taken care of? What about the snow in the driveway, turning off the water valve? What if the power goes out near your house and there's no heat?...and on and on and on.

Our everyday lives are so routine we don't stop and think of all the things that need to be done, attended to, worked on. We don't focus on them until we're not there and then it's "whoa." Your life will no longer be routine once you enter into a transplant program. It can't be. Think about it; what were once small, insignificant problems, will all of a sudden loom large if not paid attention to. Daunting and scary—yes, but you can and will get through it with help.

Side note:

When it comes to family, there's an old saying, "You can pick your friends and you can pick your nose, but you can't pick your family." Whether this saying is appropriate for your family situation or not, I don't know, but family can, may, could—emphasis on all three—be a problem. You want to tread lightly when asking certain family members for help because they might take you up on it.

Let's just say you have an imaginary brother who is currently out of work. Mr. Imaginary might visit your hospital room all day long so he can watch reruns of *Duck Dynasty* and eat leftover hospital food. You laugh, but this could be your state of affairs if you're not careful. You might wake up one morning to see imaginary little cousin Jimmy, who is no longer little, with a purple Mohawk unloading his broken-down, 1975 Volkswagen van on the street level because he's been living "down by the river" and figures he can camp in your hospital room to "help out." Sadie, who spends her days protesting marijuana laws and the killing of rats, could move in your home's guest bedroom and have smokin' parties. Johnnycakes from Kentucky, who has a tobacco chew addiction, might come over a few days a week to wait for you to fall asleep so he can quickly down some of your fun Norco pills. Hey, I'm just sayin'. Probably wouldn't happen...could, though....I mean...well...probably won't? Maybe?

It's like this. The Saturday Night Live skit "Drunk Uncle" isn't fantasy. It originated from family gatherings worldwide that went wrong. Over drinking, bad timing on voiced opinions, political arguments, Aunt Harriet's sickeningly sweet perfume fumigating the dining room on Thanksgiving, cousin Ronnie throwing a real brick at your brand new TV because the Lions lost—again, Margie falling asleep in her mashed potatoes—again, or a shaved-head teenage grandson with spikes and tats all over his face expounding on the merits of his cult.

Be careful and smart. Family matters can come back and haunt you.

On the really big other hand, you might be able to get closer to a family member you haven't spent time with in years. Bobbie's daughter Alycia might turn out to be the nicest human bean in the world and a great checkers player. Your cousin George might help you out financially when you never expected it. Other cousin Johnny, who is a doctor, might keep in constant touch with you explaining different and confusing hospital procedures, meds, and continually keeping your "dabbers up." Your mom and dad, who throughout your life should have won the Mom and Dad of the Year Award, might end up being exactly what you needed: a wonderful, loving mom and dad who would do anything to make you ok and happy.

The point is, no matter how your family/friends are involved, what is going on with you is going to affect them. It will affect them far more than you think. We know people love us. We say, "Luv you" quickly every day on the phone or when we leave the house looking back at our daughter or partner, waving. They say it back and it's nice, really nice. But the reality is their deep love for you is in jeopardy, in turmoil. They know you may not make it through surgery. They understand the consequences. They don't talk about it, but they know. Don't think they don't. It's on their mind all day long, just as it is with you. The effects of your unknown future can press their hearts and manifest themselves in strange behavior, excessive worry, frustration, sleepless nights, or problems at work or with their marriage.

Personally, I never saw one particular family issue coming. All the while I was trying hard to be positive each day, to get through the next test, to not be a bother, my emphasis was on myself. It wasn't narcissism. It seemed if I just worked at being a great patient, my chances of survival would increase and it would help my family cope. Good things would happen, I'd be okay, and possibly live many more years with my family. Doing so was for myself and my family—together. All of us. I tried for them and made it my top priority, my entire focus.

Whilst concentrating on putting in as much effort as I could to get better, I lost track of how deeply my family was being affected. My daughter and I, as mentioned earlier, are very close. Being an only child, Zachera had no siblings to fall back on during the days her father was on the brink of possibly dying. Yes, she had her mom, but her mom was in total positive mode, no matter what happened. She had to be. There was no shaking her. Jackie was completely locked on to the idea that if we both stayed positive, if everyone around us stayed positive, if the pizza delivery guy was positive, we would be ok.

Whether it was a good thing or not, Jackie never talked about negative things. She absolutely would—not—do it. Nohow, no way. In her mind she was willing me better, and that was that. Some would say it isn't healthy to put up a wall against the reality of any situation. May be true in many cases, but in Jackie's mind, I would get better if we both stayed positive and never ever discussed the negative. Did it work? Undeniably. There were hundreds of factors as to why I had such a successful transplant, but I truly believe Jackie's positive mode was one of the top reasons. It carried us thr ough.

But, as things in life go, the same mental state wasn't happening with Zachera. As days wore on during my recovery, it became clear my daughter had struggled greatly with what was going to happen during the months leading up to my transplant. Even when I was recovering, she wasn't getting any better. She had trouble with her work, she spent an inordinate amount of time with us at the hospital trying to help in some way, she became obsessed with every single directive my doctors gave me. She was extremely stressed, saying things like, "Dadddd! You have to take your pills exactly when they tell you!" or "Dadddd! You can't eat that; it's not on your list!" She was sometimes curt, wasn't happy, and seemed angry.

Looking back, it made sense. But hindsight is a set of numbers and Zachera's inner health regarding having me die was truly off track. Her backstory was different than most. No one ever got seriously sick in our family, and my parents died when she was a baby, so she never went through that experience. Jackie's parents were healthy as could be and in their nineties. No relatives died. Even her dog is healthy and going to live to be eighty-five. Zachera never experienced death, and then it was knocking on her dad's doorstep.

Interestingly, Zachera came close to dying when she was fourteen. She was in a near life-ending accident, broke six ribs, suffered a concussion, a punctured lung, and a severed liver. For five days ICU doctors in her children's hospital in Grand Rapids, Michigan, couldn't tell us whether she would live or die. They just told us the only thing they could: "Time will tell." After fighting hard to stay alive and going through grueling months of recovery, Zachera made it back. Whether this caused mental issues dealing with my transplant, I don't know. My guess, it did.

One thing I do know for sure, my daughter knows me in and out. She knows I'm terrible at following directions, eat what I want when I want, order double pepperoni on my pizza even with a wire up my nose, double dip, don't work out consistently, and lift things I'm not supposed to.

She would always joke when I would exhibit one of these famous qualities, "You're a rebel without a cause, Dad."

This was all fine and good during normal business hours—a.k.a. life—but it doesn't work so well when you're lying in a hospital bed with tubes coming out of your body from every direction. Then, throw in battling an extremely serious disease. I know Jackie harbored the same emotions inside, but never, ever let them out. Zachera, on the other hand, always wore her emotions on her right embroidered sleeve, as they say.

Thus, Zachera had many deep reasons and *modus operandi* for creating worry, stress, distress, and SOS signals about my behavior/situation. As it turned out, what she was doing wasn't always the best thing for me, even though she was trying as hard as she could to love me. Recovery was stressful—Zachera got stressed—I got stressed from her stress—then she'd stress some more. Jackie would get upset, I'd get frustrated, and, one day, the bag of uncooked spaghetti ended up in little pieces on the floor. We were all trying to do the best we could with the circumstances, but we weren't in sync.

After having a long, loud, exhausting discussion, which eventually needed to happen, Zachera and I calmed down. Things were at a standstill. A pause ensued. Then another one. Finally, I said, "Zachera, ask me what I need."

Zachera said, "I don't really want to talk about this anymore."

I came back with, "Oh, don't even do that."

She said, "Fineeee...what do you mean?"

"I mean, ask me what I need—don't tell me what I need. The

nurses are doing a fine job of telling me what I need. So, ask me right now."

"Dad, this is ridiculous."

"No, it's not. Ask me."

With a frown, she asked me, "Okayyy, what do you need?"

"I've realized, when things get difficult, I need you to walk beside me, not in front of me. You want to help me so badly and want me to have a successful recovery, to live a long, long time. But that's my job. I will be better at it if you walk beside me, encourage me, make me laugh, cry with me, and hold me up. Walking in front of me, trying to pave the way, is the doctors' and nurses' job. I don't want it to be your job. I just need you beside me, holding my hand."

She looked deeply at me and let out a long, overdue sigh. We cried some and hugged a good long time. Zachera finally let go and said, "I've been overdoing it...I know...a lot...but it's only because I love you and want you to be ok."

"I know...and I understand." Lots of emotions.

Jackie put plates on the table filled with new spaghetti she made in a crock pot on the small, two-foot Formica hotel counter. (I don't recommend making spaghetti in a crock pot. It's nasty, but it was the only way we could cook without smoke wafting up into the hotel's alarm and having five helmeted Chicago firemen burst into our room with axes in hand.) Jackie kept us.

Moral of the story: talk to each other, be honest with each other, and be aware that the people around you may have problems dealing with the whole damn thing. People always say, "Communication is key." Well, some clichés are true. The English professor expounds, "Avoid the dreaded cliché." In this case, use them all you want.

All the loving and caring matters. My mom and dad passed away ten years before I came down with IPF. They were wonderful, loving parents. Jackie, Zachera, and Ryan were by my side throughout my initial IPF prognoses, my innumerable testing, the waiting for the donor call, the rushing to the hospital for my transplant, the sleeping in an extremely cold pre-surgery room, the waiting all night for me to finally head into surgery, my long recovery, and life ever after. Jackie's mom and dad, who are in their nineties, kept in touch the best way they could from northern Michigan and encouraged all of us at every turn. They even made the trip down to Chicago from Boyne City to see me, even though it was very difficult for them. My friends visited, taking me to dinner at a special restaurant downtown and watching over our house in the northern woods during our four-month stay next to MMHMMM. They all made my days cheerful, loving, and positive. What else could I have asked for? My family, my friends, and my medical staff all took care of me. That's why I'm here.

27

When All is Said and Done

Headed home! Yay!!! Breakfast with Zachera and Ryan, packed up and headed to northern Michigan! Stopped by Boyne Mountain for dinner as we got close. Drove down our tree-lined drive-way, saw yellow ribbons tied to some trees, and a big "Welcome Home!" sign on our garage door. It was all Dad's doing, and Mom had placed a beautiful bouquet of white calla lilies at our door! I got out and hugged the corner of my house. It had been a long, long, long five months. Inside there were flowers and Su's gorgeous painted swan. Our house seemed so large after being in a hotel room for so many months. I stood there and looked and looked. As we unpacked, it was clear I had way too many clothes in my closet. We learned how to live simply and with no room. Time to clean out and downsize! This whole experience has shed lots of light. We learned so much and we're home!! – Jac

Today, sitting here at my desk writing…breathing in and out…I celebrate my life. I do it every day. My deep, deep smile emanates from a boy on the streets of Detroit, the night my Dad watched me play in our high-school championship football game, when Jackie walked down the aisle to marry me, the night my mother and I said goodbye as she died in my arms, when Jackie gave me our baby daughter and Zachera looked up into my eyes for the first time.

My smile also comes from the moment incredible doctors told me I was breathing on my own after having someone else's lungs placed inside me. All along the way, I have been, as Lou Gehrig said, "the luckiest man on the face of the earth." Magnificently lucky is the only phrase to explain my days dancing in this world. Robin Williams told us in *Dead Poet's Society* to go out and make our lives extraordinary. Standing on my chair, I told him I tried.

My lung transplant experience turned out to be extraordinary. It was wild, like the Mousetrap amusement ride at Edgewater Park in Detroit. I was the kid who never wanted the ride to end, but when it did, remembered every single second forever.

I keep saying my lung transplant seemed "out of time"—separated from the rest of my life. I don't think that sensation will ever change. It happened. It just seems so strange that I went...and came back.

But I'm here writing in my den. I'm here...in northern Michigan. In my home. I have new lungs. When I go to bed, they breathe for me. Waking up in the cool, crisp morning, they take in air and send oxygenated blood to my heart to propel throughout my body. Every breath a miraculous conversion. When I ride my bike up a long, steep hill, my new lungs work hard and billow and help take me to my destination. I can laugh with friends without coughing, talk without running out of breath, and do so many of the things I couldn't do seven or eight years ago.

Most important of all...I can continue loving Jackie, who is, to me, the most incredibly strong and devoted person in the world. The day Jackie and I met changed my life. We went to see the movie *Wonder Woman* the other night and all through the movie I felt strange because Wonder Woman was sitting right next to me. If it hadn't been for Jackie, I would not have made it back...would not be sitting here writing this. Truly, Jackie allowed positive, lucky patterns to surround and guide me. I will always, always love her and promise to meet her, third star on the left and straight on 'til morning.

Thanks to many, many phenomenal human beings at MMHMMM,

I can continue to love my daughter because I'm here. I have the days to do so. I can boast about her career, can watch her grow, enjoy her strength and fortitude, marvel at her love for her husband Ryan, appreciate the art she creates, and feel ecstatic every day about bringing her into this world. She, too, is making her life extraordinary.

I can constantly marvel at Ryan's will and intelligence, watch his career grow, and drink a beer with a man who will forever be my son. We can go to a ballgame at Wrigley Field, root for our college team, cook splendid dinners, have him fix my cellphone, and visit out-of-the-way ethnic restaurants in strong-shouldered Chicago. I can feel restful inside knowing Zachera found an excellent man with whom to spend her life.

If I could, I'd share all my outcomes with the wonderful people I met along my transplant journey. The people who were experiencing a transplant next to me, who were spending the same days. If I could just share my fortune with all the people who received a transplant or are about to—those incredibly strong, tough patients. I was constantly in awe of those around me who fought every day to stay alive. How they endured incredible discomfort and the darkest of odds. How they turned their faces towards their problem, not away. How they bravely said yes to whatever procedure a doctor needed to do because, as my hospital roommate would say, "livin' better than dyin'." They never gave up, they never gave in, they kept on keeping on.

It would be wonderful to tell you each and every one of their stories. They are libraries holding stories needing to be told. Heroic stories. That's why the hospital staff calls them heroes. Each person is special within their own walk on Earth—characters in their moment of time. Some didn't make it simply because their bodies wouldn't let them go any farther. Unfortunately, we can't live forever. It was sad for all of us when someone didn't make it. We wanted them to keep on so badly.

While getting me ready to be discharged from the hospital, one of my nurses said, "You're a hero." I was taken back and quizzically asked, "Why do you say that?"

"Because you are," she countered. "You made it through the toughest and largest surgery there is. You are living with transplanted lungs. Only heroes can do that."

Looking down at the floor, I immediately said, "I'm not a hero. I appreciate you saying that, but so many people helped me." My mind raced to how lucky I was, to all the patients who had it tougher, harder, who endured depressingly difficult moments that would try any person's heart and soul. I thought about the cancer patients on the floor below me, about visiting them—about walking those halls with ten-year-old Arielle. How difficult their condition was because they never really knew, even when their doctors had hope, if they were cured, never knew if their cancer would come roaring back.

Looking up at the nurse, I said, "It's just that...I was so lucky. While I was here, I met a teacher who donated one of her kidneys so her young cousin could live. She's the hero. I met a patient who was having his fifteenth operation to fix a mysterious disease the doctors couldn't figure out. How could someone get through all that? I asked him, 'What's keeping you going?' His reply, 'I want them to find a cure for this damn thing so if someone else gets it, they'll be able to save 'em.' He's the hero."

No matter what happened, no matter how hard it was, the patients I met along the way never went "gently into the night." I salute them all. They fought to keep on living. They tried to stay for the people who loved them no matter what. They did it so they could walk their daughter down the aisle at her wedding, so they could sit on the end of the dock fishing with their grandson, or to stroll, one more time, down to their mailbox inhaling...inhaling deeply the crisp scent of autumn on the dawn of a beautiful new morning.

Afterword

Experiences teach. After living through momentous events, you come away with important lessons learned. What were my lessons? To sum them all up would take pages and pages, so here are my Top Ten Transplant Lessons, in no particular order:

1. Recognize when you are kind to others, it multiplies. Organ donors give life. Prized life. Insanely powerful life. One of the most giving decisions a person can make is to donate a viable organ to another human being after someone has died, or, in some cases, while a person is still living. Please try to understand the incredible impact of organ donation.

2. Going on a serious health journey sends you on a special hospital ride called, borrowing from our friends The Beatles, The Magical Mystery Tour. Once on this rollercoaster, strap in, sit back, and take off full force with a smile on your face. There's absolutely no reason to delve into self-pity, anger, or resentment: "Why did this have to happen to me?" Well, it did. Get on with it and do your best. Understand this is for you, and also for your loved ones.

3. There's an incredible life force within us. It's the force powering survival. Meeting this force face-to-face gives us the energy and force to keep on keeping on. Patients next to me at MMHMMM went through whatever it took to keep going. You could see this force in their eyes, especially when a loved one stood next to their bedside. It's strong. Embrace it. Others choose to let their life fade away, which is their decision and no one else's. There are times that

decision is best. We are not on this earth to suffer endlessly. It's not a choice in which anyone should ever pass judgment. It's the most personal and private decision you will ever make—to live on or die. Hopefully you'll know when the time comes. If you aren't capable mentally or physically to know or make that decision—that's a whole different discussion. But please, if it's time to fight on—fight on. If it's time to let go—let go. Your call, no one else's. I've been on the brink—it's powerful.

4. Frozen soup can be heated up again. There really are re-dos in this world. Never ever forget you can find a way around roadblocks. Not always, but more times than you would ever think. This not only applies to your health, but to life itself. Throughout your days on this planet, there will be roadblocks—fight around them. "Do not go quietly into the night."

5. Caring for another person here on Earth is the pinnacle of love. Nothing is higher. You may go through life surrounded by other possible achievements, but loving and caring for the ones you love will always be number one on the AP poll. Quote me on that. You can have all the riches, fame, and glory in the world, but when your life comes down to it, how much you loved—truly loved—will be the difference.

6. Good people make our lives. People who care only for themselves and no one else are forgotten and become dust in the wind. Good people live on…in others.

7. It's the little things. We hear that all the time only because it's true. Whilst I was being interviewed about this book, a columnist asked, "Can you elaborate on some big things that happened during your transplant?" My answer: "In retrospect, it was an accumulation of little things. Yes, breathing on my own after my transplant was big…more than big. But it truly was the little things that counted: the nurse who helped me into a comfortable

position in bed when my whole body hurt; the gurney driver who tried to cheer me up with his son's favorite joke; Jackie being there to give me another blanket—always, always being there for me; bendable straws; friends visiting from my little town; a doctor who really cared; fuzzy blue hospital socks with knobby, non-slip soles; a daughter staying mentally parallel when I needed her the most; shower chairs; blue Jiffy Pop hats making me laugh; Ryan being a rock in every situation; pictures of their dog Oliver sleeping upside down on his beanbag. The list could go on and on." Big things are made up of little things along the way.

8. Realize how talented surgeons really are, what it took to gain their knowledge, and what they go through day after day to save lives. In the morning they attempt to save a person's life—then, they do it again after lunch.

9. You've heard strength comes from within. Well, others can help, but whether you are going to live or die—is all you. When the lights go out for the night and the only sound in your hospital room is the low hum of a machine keeping you alive, you are at your core—the deep inside. That's where your answer resides.

10. Know that loving others and being a good person on our earth matters.

Thanks for listening,
Em

Author's Bio

Robert Emmet was born in Detroit in 1950 – then a city of street hockey, sandlot baseball, and touch football with parked cars as end zones. He watched Gordie Howe and the Detroit Red Wings in the Stanley Cup Finals, and followed a winning Detroit Lions football team.

After college, he and wife Jackie moved to northern Michigan. She taught first grade while Robert taught high school English. They also co-directed the theater program at Boyne City Schools for 40 years.

Emmet has been a writer, artist, truck driver, carpenter, tour guide, and multi-sports coach. His work has touched, he says, "hundreds and hundreds of incredible students who made my life extraordinary."

Adds the author: "Cat Stevens once wrote, 'We only dance upon this Earth a short while....' Well, I've danced."

Made in the USA
Middletown, DE
28 July 2020